"The Bittersweet Farm Model is really effective for individuals with severe sensory problems, aggressive behavior, and intellectual disability. The emphasis on farm life, sensory rich activity, and physical labor is calming."

—Temple Grandin, author, *The Autistic Brain*

"While many have elected to live and work in rural America, the options for adults with autism to pursue a similar lifestyle were nearly non-existent. Yet, the pleasures of working the land, caring for animals, and appreciating the change of seasons can become the backdrop for supporting and engaging everyone, including those with autism.

Bittersweet began as a dream. It is a dream shared by many families, but few have succeeded at making that dream a reality. As adults with autism have struggled to find homes and communities that recognize their unique perspective and contributions, the founders of Bittersweet unified a collection of leaders and resources to find creative solutions. Individuals with autism, families and professionals will each find something in the Bittersweet vision. Learn from their journey and pick up valuable practical examples by reading this book."

—Steven Muller, CEO, Balance Autism

"As the grandfather of two young adults with autism, I found this book really valuable—a must read to learn how to help provide meaning and purpose to those on the spectrum ... and to benefit yourself from a loving relationship."

—Bill Novelli, professor, McDonough School of Business, Georgetown University and former CEO, AARP

"Bittersweet Farms is widely admired for the quality and depth of their programs that embrace individuality. This book provides valuable insight into creating a purposeful community where adults with autism can live, work, and flourish."

—Ashley Kim Weiss, executive director for Together For Choice, an advocacy organization aimed at promoting the spectrum of housing/service models for people with autism and other developmental disabilities

"Bittersweet represents the ideal autism service provider. Their personalized, respectful approach focuses on functional meaningful activities in a natural environment. Both on the farm and within the larger community, Bittersweet offers its participants acceptance, purpose and belonging. It is exactly what this doctor recommends!"

—Karen Ratliff-Schaub, MD, MBOE, medical director, developmental pediatrics, program director, developmental behavioral pediatric fellowship and Prisma Health Children's Hospital–Upstate, Greenville, South Carolina

"I am happy to support this book describing the Bittersweet Farms model for meeting the complex needs of adults with autism. The book clearly outlines the benefits of care farming for adults with disabilities and is sure to be an invaluable guide for programs in other communities. As a parent of a young adult with autism spectrum disorder and as a director of a nature-based program for youth and young adults with disabilities, I am aware of the benefits of farming and nature for all, but particularly for people with differing abilities."

—Lisa Burris, executive director, Turn Back Time (a farm and nature-focused program for children in Paxton, Massachusetts)

"From its inception, Bittersweet Farms was envisioned as a therapeutic community where those with autism could continue to grow and flourish as adults. Those of us on staff and the families knew it succeeded in providing that and more. A good quality of life was always the goal, individualized for each person. Until Dr Dennler took on the project of analyzing and evaluating data and other aspects of the residents' lives, we did not have the empirical evidence to validate what we knew intuitively. Professionals and families traveled to Bittersweet from all over the world, seeking to understand how to replicate a program that would accomplish this goal. Now with this book, many more can understand the concepts Bittersweet was built on."

—Vickie Obee, former director of Bittersweet Farms

Creating Quality of Life for Adults on the Autism Spectrum

Creating Quality of Life for Adults on the Autism Spectrum: The Story of Bittersweet Farms provides an overview of the first farmstead community for adults with autism established in North America. The book also provides a detailed description and evaluation of the intervention model used to promote quality of life for the adults with autism who live as residents at Bittersweet Farms.

Through its aim to provide a better understanding of adults with autism spectrum disorder (ASD), the text enables a deeper appreciation of the Bittersweet Farms model, which meets the residential and therapeutic needs of this population that are not often well understood. The book discusses the apprenticeship model used at Bittersweet Farms along with examples of how residents benefit from this approach. The text expands upon its approach through the inclusion of specific guidelines that can be adopted for improved communication and social interaction, managing troublesome behaviors, calming anxieties, and establishing daily routines. These guidelines reflect a positive approach to intervention and are consistent with the quality-of-life emphasis inherent in the Bittersweet model.

This book will serve as a seminal work for professionals and paraprofessionals working with people with ASD. It will further be of interest to parents and relatives of people with ASD along with researchers and policymakers concerned about the ASD adult population, and those interested in services for people with ASD.

Jeanne Dennler is a retired clinical psychologist with over 40 years working in private practice as a psychologist specializing in children and adults with autism, and has published numerous articles in professional journals. She served on the board of Bittersweet Farms and is a former clinical assistant professor of pediatrics, Division of Developmental and Behavioral Pediatrics.

Carol S. Quick worked as a special education teacher, administrator, and director of varied federal and state-funded early intervention projects. Her professional writing accomplishments include the production of professional development modules, grant proposals, and evaluation plans. She has also served as a board member and consultant for numerous disability-focused organizations.

Ruth Wilson has authored several academic books, including *Special Educational Needs in the Early Years* (Routledge, 2003), *Nature and Young Children* (Routledge, 2018), and *Naturally Inclusive* (Gryphon House, 2022). She currently works with the Children & Nature Network as curator of the research library.

Creating Quality of Life for Adults on the Autism Spectrum

The Story of Bittersweet Farms

Jeanne Dennler, Carol S. Quick and Ruth Wilson

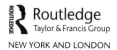

Routledge
Taylor & Francis Group

NEW YORK AND LONDON

Cover image: Getty Images

First published 2023
by Routledge
605 Third Avenue, New York, NY 10158

and by Routledge
4 Park Square, Milton Park, Abingdon, Oxon, OX14 4RN

Routledge is an imprint of the Taylor & Francis Group, an informa business

Library of Congress Cataloging-in-Publication Data
Names: Dennler, Jeanne, author. | Quick, Carol S., author. |
Wilson, Ruth A., 1943- author.
Title: Creating quality of life for adults on the autism spectrum : the story
of Bittersweet Farms / Jeanne Dennler, Carol S. Quick, Ruth Wilson.
Description: New York, NY : Routledge, 2023. | Includes bibliographical
references and index. |
Identifiers: LCCN 2022015832 (print) | LCCN 2022015833 (ebook)
| ISBN 9781032220642 (hbk) | ISBN 9781032220628 (pbk) |
ISBN 9781003271048 (ebk)
Subjects: LCSH: Autistic people. | Autism--Treatment. | Bittersweet
Farms (Ohio) | Quality of life.
Classification: LCC HV1570.23 .D46 2023 (print) | LCC HV1570.23
(ebook) | DDC 616.85/882--dc23/eng/20220706
LC record available at https://lccn.loc.gov/2022015832
LC ebook record available at https://lccn.loc.gov/2022015833

ISBN: 9781032220642 (hbk)
ISBN: 9781032220628 (pbk)
ISBN: 9781003271048 (ebk)

DOI: 10.4324/9781003271048

Typeset in Bembo
by Deanta Global Publishing Services, Chennai, India

To the Bittersweet families who have worked so tirelessly to provide quality of life for their children!

Contents

Foreword

For as long as we can remember, our son has loved farms. This is nothing unusual for severely autistic guys (and gals) like Ben. The farmer, the farmer's wife, and especially, the animals and all of the activities surrounding them—kids' farm videos and books would hold him in rapt attention. And now, at 28, they still do.

My wife Karen and I used to say that Ben would be in heaven if he could live on a farm, the real thing. It seemed like an almost magical, mystical idea, a farm with a caring and dedicated staff delivering the services he needed, safe and sound, along with farmers and farm animals.

Then we thought, hey, maybe we could put something like that together for Ben! Of course, ideas are fun and easy. The actual implementation? Five minutes with Google looking at farms brought us back to reality.

And then Google presented us with exactly what we were imagining—Bittersweet Farms. We were stunned.

Here was a place that not only offered what we had imagined, but went so far beyond it that we had to see it for ourselves.

I have often thought that one of the few positives about Ben's autism is the extraordinary people we have gotten to know because of it: therapists, caregivers, doctors, families, others like us, moving through the world of autism.

Like Vicki Obee. If anyone in the world personified the kind of extraordinary people you can meet in the world of autism, it is Vicki. Now retired, when we first spoke, she was executive director of Bittersweet Farms.

The day after our Googled discovery of Bittersweet, we were on the phone with Vicki, a warm, sympathetic, smart, funny, resourceful, problem-solving, and welcoming soul, who invited us over to take a look. Whitehouse, Ohio, near Toledo, is an easy drive from Chicago, our home base at the time. A week later, we arrived at Bittersweet Farms.

As we got out of the car, our first impression was that Bittersweet was, well, a farm. Nothing struck us as out of the ordinary. There were fields, barns, animals, hoop houses (a type of greenhouse, we city slickers later learned), people doing what looked like farm stuff (more city slicker terminology), but there was nothing to suggest that the place was anything special.

Just a farm.

By the time we left, we were blown away.

This book will show you why.

Along with learning about autism itself, you will discover a program that addresses one of the biggest needs in the world of severe autism—services for adults impacted by the disorder. In the media, we usually hear only about the children and young people with autism. What we don't see are these people, 20, 30, 40 years later.

This is a population that is exploding. The severe autism "epidemic" is very real. These are people who simply cannot live—survive—independently, for so many reasons.

That is *not* to say that they cannot be independent within a system that supports their likes, desires, abilities, strengths, and the things that they enjoy and make them happy, and yes, fulfilled.

Bittersweet is that extremely rare kind of place. It has served as a model for many other programs that have appeared in the years and decades since it was founded by an extraordinary, brilliant, pioneering, and hugely inspirational powerhouse named Bettye Ruth. Almost a half-century ago, she saw a need, and saw one way to address it. And that was only the beginning.

She, and Bittersweet, and everything that has happened over the past half-century, make for quite a story, and we are lucky that the person telling that story is Jeanne Dennler. Actually, she is *Doctor* Jeanne Dennler, a psychologist who knows autism, knows Bittersweet, and knows how important it is to get the Bittersweet story out there. Bittersweet has already inspired others to follow its lead in creating farmsteads in their own parts of the world. The leaders of Bittersweet have always been eager to share their vast knowledge and experience with any and all who might want practical advice on how to do it.

And this book is the next step on that mission—to inspire and instruct others on how to follow their lead. It is not simply a feel-good story—though I promise, you will often feel, not just good, but inspired as you read it, not always the case with autism. It is informative and based on current, cutting-edge research.

In other words, in a sphere where there are many more questions than answers, Bittersweet is what the world of autism needs, right now, more than ever.

Because nobody's getting any younger.

David Royko is a clinical psychologist, mediator, writer, husband of Karen, and father of Jake and Ben. His writing on autism has appeared in many places including the *Chicago Tribune*, *Chicago Parent*, *Parents Magazine*, and his blog: The Chronicles of Ben: Autism in Real Time.

—David Royko, PsyD

Endorsement

Bittersweet Farms represents a rare and important resource for people interested in understanding the experiences of a diverse group of autistic adults across the lifespan. Only a few service providers in the world have focused exclusively on the autistic adult population for as long as Bittersweet: nearly 40 years of developing and refining autism-informed programs of support and life enrichment.

The autistic men and women of Bittersweet range from young adults to seniors. Their support needs are moderate through intense. Their backgrounds are diverse. They came to Bittersweet from family homes, group homes, state institutions, and independent living settings, all unable to help them lead happy, safe, and fulfilling lives. But each found support, and thrived, at Bittersweet. It's an amazing success story. The terrific autistic adults you'll learn about have much to teach the world, as do Bittersweet's leaders and staff, both past and present. I hope you'll join me in reading Dr Jeanne Dennler's in-depth exploration of Bittersweet Farms.

Every year, people from around the country and the world travel to Bittersweet in Whitehouse, Ohio (just outside Toledo), to learn about the holistic and healthy work/live model that this intentional community embraces. Many arrive with the idea of replicating the Bittersweet model close to home. Some start by saying, "I found this beautiful farm." But most discover that reproducing Bittersweet involves far more than acquiring an idyllic farm. Rather, it's the relationship between the holistic support model and setting that's the secret to Bittersweet's success. Bittersweet is not isolated. The people, both residents and staff, and their farm operations, which include a community supported agricultural (CSA) program, are all strongly, and undeniably, woven into the fabric of their broader community.

In recent years, spurred on by the landmark US Supreme Court Olmstead decision and state-based deinstitutionalization efforts, elected officials, public policymakers, advocacy organizations, families, and advocates, including self-advocates, have been engaged in a welcome effort to restructure the system of supports and services for intellectual and developmentally disabled Americans, including autistic adults. This restructuring, sometimes referred to as rebalancing, prioritizes the development and funding of integrated community-based service and support infrastructure over historic, large-scale congregate care models.

The founder of Bittersweet Farms, Bettye Ruth Kay, a progressive special education teacher in the Toledo, Ohio school system, knew that the archaic institutional system was poorly designed for autistic adults. She saw the bleak, and dangerous, future of institutional placement that awaited many of her students after they aged out of school-based entitlements. Ms Kay created and developed Bittersweet as an alternative to segregated, large-scale institutional congregate care models, which included involuntary, rural, state-run industrial farms for intellectual and developmentally disabled adults. Her vision was to help "autistic people (grow) in every area of life, using the rural, extended family community as the model."

Sadly, some leading disability rights advocates insist on conflating Bittersweet, and similar voluntary intentional community models, with large, involuntary 19th-century institutions, despite overwhelming evidence to the contrary. Unfortunately, this inaccurate and unfair notion has created policy and economic barriers to the replication of Bittersweet's inclusive model, though some notable exceptions do exist. I hope that Dr Dennler's work helps correct this unfair narrative, so that the thousands of autistic adults who want a holistic provider model and supportive community like Bittersweet can enjoy the same positive outcomes and life experiences that you'll learn about in this book.

—Gene Bensinger

Gene Bensinger is a managing director in institutional sales at Mesirow Financial, a diversified financial services firm headquartered in Chicago. Gene has been a leading national advocate on a wide range of autism-related issues for over 20 years.

Gene helped lead the successful coalition-based effort to enact autism insurance reform in Illinois from 2004 to 2007. In 2008, he helped create, and served on the advisory committee for, the Autism Speaks Autism Safety Project. Gene also participated in President Barack Obama's inaugural White House conference on autism in 2011. From 2014 to 2017, Gene worked with a bipartisan coalition of legislators to help create landmark ABLE Savings Plans, which are similar to college savings plans for people with a wide range of disabilities who meet certain qualifications.

Currently, Gene is working closely with national, state, and local policymakers, advocates, and elected officials on autism-related policy and legislation around the issues of housing, employment, safety, adult supports and services, and financial security. He regularly speaks on these topics to groups at conferences and events.

Gene formerly served on the Autism Speaks Chicagoland Chapter Board. Gene and his wife, Lynn Straus, live in Chicago and have two adult sons, the eldest of whom is profoundly autistic.

Introduction

The Introduction provides a brief description of Bittersweet Farms and the farmstead model. It presents a compelling discussion in support of Bittersweet Farms and the farmstead model as an appropriate setting for adults with autism spectrum disorder (ASD). The Introduction also provides a general description of autism, an overview of the book, and a brief introduction to several major concepts discussed later in the book. These concepts include quality of life, eco-psychosomatics, neurodiversity, and sensory processing. Research relating to each of these concepts is presented and discussed. The Bittersweet model, as described in the Introduction, recognizes that ASD is a lifelong condition presenting special challenges for individuals with this condition. The model is based on the understanding that interventions in the form of a supportive environment can improve the quality of life for individuals with ASD.

Bittersweet vines grow on the property of Bittersweet Farms in Ohio. Other things grow there, too—trees, tomatoes, lettuce, farm animals, and the spirits of the people who live and work on this 80-acre farmstead in Whitehouse, Ohio. The small village of Whitehouse is surrounded by farm country, and from the outside, Bittersweet Farms doesn't look all that different from the other farms in the area. A closer look, however, reveals the uniqueness of what Bittersweet Farms has to offer.

What is Bittersweet Farms?

Bittersweet Farms is home to adults with autism spectrum disorder (ASD) who need daily living support to realize their full range of capabilities. Living and working on the farm give residents abundant opportunities for self-paced, meaningful activities. Dedicated staff, who live and work with the residents, understand that each person with ASD is an individual with his or her own set of skills and interests. Daily activities for each resident are planned around this understanding.

DOI: 10.4324/9781003271048-1

In addition to the residential services, Bittersweet Farms also provides a range of educational and consulting services to address a variety of needs of adolescents and adults with ASD. These services are designed to increase autonomy and self-reliance, empower the ability to make choices, maximize dignity, and encourage interaction. The Bittersweet model framing each of these services is grounded in an understanding of autism, which recognizes that each individual with ASD has unique needs and special gifts.

What is Autism?

Autism is a developmental disability caused by a neurological dysfunction. While every person with ASD is a unique individual, people with autism share similar neurodevelopmental conditions which impact the way the brain performs in areas of communication skills and social interaction. These conditions lead to characteristic and predictable patterns of thinking and behavior in individuals with ASD (Mesibov et al., 2004). The communication deficit makes it difficult for many people with ASD to initiate and/or sustain a conversation. The social interaction impairments tend to manifest as failure to use eye contact and may involve unusual facial expressions. Other characteristics often seen in people with ASD include becoming intensely absorbed in a particular object, repeating motor movements over and over, and engaging in non-functional routines. Nine out of ten people with ASD also experience sensory processing problems.

Sensory processing is the ability to feel and understand sensory data from the environment and from one's own body. An individual with a sensory processing disorder may not be able to regulate the information he or she receives from the senses and thus has trouble adapting to the everyday sensations that most people take for granted. This concern is discussed in more detail in Chapters 5 and 6.

Autism is described as a "spectrum disorder" because people with autism have characteristics that fall into a spectrum, from relatively mild to very severe. The severity of the condition is based on social communication impairments and restricted, repetitive patterns of behavior. Differences in IQ account for a great deal of this variability. Temperament, interests, and unique skill patterns also make a difference. The degree of severity affects how a person with ASD communicates and interacts with the world.

Discussions about ASD often highlight deficiencies and a search for interventions to minimize the deficiencies. Some researchers and practitioners, however, advocate a different approach. They call for replacing the deficiency-oriented framework with new thinking and new terminology focusing on the strengths of individuals with ASD. Consistent with this new thinking is the idea of referring to persons with ASD as being neurodiverse instead of deficient; and instead of trying to "fix the problem," efforts focus on creating a supportive environment where capabilities and strengths are maximized (Armstrong, 2017; Robertson, 2010). Because people with autism differ from "neurotypical people," they need understanding and support to help them function well in their daily lives. That's what the Bittersweet model is all about. Bittersweet Farms was founded on the realization that many adults with ASD "generally do not function well without individualized support services that recognize their idiosyncratic style of understanding their environments, learning, and behaving" (Mesibov et al., 2004, p. 159).

The Bittersweet model recognizes that ASD is a lifelong condition presenting special challenges for individuals with this disability. The model is based on the understanding, however, that interventions in the form of a supportive environment can improve the quality of life (QOL) for individuals with ASD.

Quality of Life and Autism

Quality of life, as defined by the World Health Organization, is "individuals' perception of their position in life, in the context of the culture and value systems in which they live and in relation to their goals, expectations, standards and concerns." As this definition indicates, quality of life clearly means more than the absence of discomfort, illness, or trauma. Quality of life is a presence, an overall feeling of well-being encompassing the physical, psychological, and social aspects of one's life. Quality of life is sometimes defined and measured in relation to eight domains: interpersonal relations, social inclusion, personal development, physical well-being, self-determination, material well-being, emotional well-being, and human and legal rights (Schalock et al., 2004). The number of QOL domains is generally considered less important than the understanding that any proposed QOL model must recognize that people know what is important to them. For adults with ASD, subjective quality of life refers to the extent to which they are satisfied with various domains of their life (Hong et al., 2016).

An enhanced quality of life is a realistic and obtainable goal for all persons, including those with ASD and other types of disabilities (Schalock et al., 2004). Adults with ASD, however, generally report significantly lower subjective quality of life than adults without ASD (Moss et al., 2017). As the severity of ASD increases, the quality of life generally decreases (Mason et al., 2018). Reports also indicate that individuals with ASD across the lifespan have poor quality of life relative to their peers with other disabilities (White et al., 2018). Some of the related research suggests that quality-of-life issues for people with ASD tend to worsen with age, especially in relation to the physical and psychological areas of their lives (Mason et al., 2018). A systematic review of the literature found that less than 20% of people with ASD enjoy "good" outcomes; almost 50% have poor or very poor outcomes (Steinhausen et al., 2016).

The difficulties in social reciprocity and communication associated with autism place individuals with ASD at particular risk for a lower quality of life, especially in the interpersonal domain. Having friends contributes to QOL in this domain, yet the friendship problems many children with ASD experience during their growing up years tend to persist into adolescence and adulthood (DaWalt et al., 2019). Social participation—another quality-of-life indicator in the interpersonal domain—is also an area of concern for many people with ASD. Adults with ASD are less likely to be involved in community groups (church, school, sports, or local government groups) compared to individuals without disabilities. Adolescents and adults with ASD are also less likely to enjoy reciprocal relationships, and tend to participate in significantly fewer social and recreational activities (DaWalt et al., 2019).

Additionally, while autism is not a mental health condition, mental health problems are common in people with ASD (Khanna et al., 2014; Robertson, 2010). This applies to people with both early and later diagnoses of their ASD status (Marriage et al., 2009). Some research shows that approximately 70%–80% of people with ASD experience mental health problems (Lever & Geurts, 2016; Simonoff et al., 2008), with depression and anxiety the most common of their mental health concerns. The rate of depression for people with ASD may be as high as 41% (Howlin, 2000). Other highly prevalent mental health problems faced by people with ASD include bipolar disorder, anxiety, obsessive-compulsive disorder, and schizophrenia (Howlin, 2000). These mental health disabilities can have an enormous impact on various quality-of-life domains.

While the rates of mental health problems in people with ASD are difficult to determine, the consequences are not. Adults with ASD who experience episodes of depression report high rates of suicidal thoughts, suicide plans, or suicide attempts (Cassidy et al., 2014; Hirvikoski & Blomqvist, 2015).

Quality of life for individuals with ASD is often an important treatment outcome; and improving their quality of life is a main objective of many interventions and social services. Adults with ASD who receive support in their lives—including support with daily living tasks, help in interacting with peers, and assistance in planning daily activities—report higher social and environmental quality of life than those not receiving such support (Mason et al., 2018). Bittersweet recognizes that adults with

ASD need—and have a right to—supportive accommodations based on their unique neurological makeup.

Significant positive predictors of quality of life for the general population include being employed, receiving support, and being in a relationship (Mason et al., 2018). Research more specific to adults with ASD found that adaptive behavior, executive functioning, and perceived informal support play significant roles in their subjective quality of life (Renty & Roeyers, 2006).

In the past, research on outcomes for adults with ASD and intellectual disabilities tended to focus on such traditional achievement indicators as maintaining employment and living independently. Many individuals with severe ASD and intellectual disabilities fared poorly based on these conventional benchmarks. More recent interventions and related research on outcomes focus on quality of life across the lifespan.

The Bittersweet model reflects an understanding of the importance of quality of life for adults with ASD and addresses, in a meaningful way, different quality-of-life domains. A discussion about these domains in relation to the Bittersweet model is presented in Chapter 7.

Support for Bittersweet Farms and the Farmstead Model

Where and how we live—as well as the stability of our living arrangements—are major contributors to our quality of life. The farmstead model is one type of community housing option specifically designed to support the needs of adults with disabilities, who are often faced with less-than-ideal living arrangements. The farmstead model is set within the context of a working farm, where residents work along with staff at tasks relevant to the care and maintenance of the grounds and the farm. While the tasks generally relate to some aspect of farm living, the primary focus of each activity is on meeting individual needs and interests. On-site vocational training opportunities at Bittersweet are varied and include horticulture, greenhouse management, woodworking, animal care, and landscaping. The farm environment and most of the vocational training activities at Bittersweet engage residents in active, hands-on engagement with the natural world.

Eco-psychosomatics

Bittersweet Farms was established before we knew much about eco-psychosomatics—that is, the study of the close connection between mind, body, and nature. This evolving field of biomedical research has a lot to say about the health-promoting effects of contact with plants, animals, and natural environments. The health-related benefits of engagement with nature apply to physical, mental, and spiritual dimensions of human health and well-being. The entire milieu of a farmstead model promotes deep engagement with the natural world and thus reflects an eco-psychosomatic view of life and health.

Eco-psychosomatics and other research on the benefits of nature for humans indicate that people tend to be happier, healthier, more socially engaged, and more creative when nature is an integral part of their daily lives (Arvay, 2018a; Bratman et al., 2019; Twohig-Bennett & Jones, 2018). These findings apply to people of all ages and abilities, including people with ASD (Li et al., 2019). Clemens Arvay, an Austrian biologist and author, is a strong advocate for an eco-psychosomatic view of life and health. His research highlights the importance of nature-human medicine (Arvay, 2018a).

In *The Healing Code of Nature*, Arvay (2018a) explains how the term "eco-psychosomatics," when first used in the 1990s, referred to the investigation of harmful environmental influences on the body and the psyche. Since then, our understanding of eco-psychosomatics has broadened. Eco-psychosomatics, as an interdisciplinary exploration of nature-human medicine, now views humans as part of the network of life and focuses on the physical and mental therapeutic effects of nature on humans. Arvay's research includes investigations into the benefits of nature for people with ASD.

People with ASD tend to experience more troublesome anxiety conditions (including generalized anxiety disorder) than other groups. Anxiety for people with ASD is often associated with increased aggression, conduct problems, depression, self-injury, insistence on sameness, and irritability (Ambler et al., 2015; Lidstone et al., 2014). Exposure to natural environments may lower stress and anxiety and potentially minimize some of the associated problematic behaviors (Barakat et al., 2019; Bratman et al., 2015; Kuo, 2015). Research shows that contact with nature evokes a positive affect, which may then block negative or stressful thoughts and feelings (Ulrich, 1983). Literature reviews confirm these findings (Masterton et al., 2020; Reyes-Riveros et al., 2021). Such reviews also indicate that contact with natural environments is associated with reductions in anger, fatigue, anxiety, and sadness (Li et al., 2019).

People with autism may find it difficult to shift attention flexibly, especially when prompted to do so by another person. There are some indications that exposure to natural environments may improve the attentional states of adults with ASD. Affordances in nature and animals may help people with autism become curious and show interest in nature-related happenings. At times, this interest then prompts positive interaction with others (Bystrom et al., 2019). This phenomenon was observed in children who were participating in a treatment program located on a small farm with animals and the surrounding natural environment. While at the farm, children engaged in such activities as horse riding, playing outdoor games, and caring for the animals. Research data collected over a period of 18 months indicated that the program was effective in reducing stress, awakening curiosity and interest, prompting spontaneous attention, and vitalizing energy. The researchers concluded that the soft and repetitive movements occurring in nature and animal behavior played a role in reducing stress and promoting calmness in the children with ASD. The researchers also noted that the children's spontaneous attention to the movement dynamics of nature and animals provided them with a higher degree of vitality and mental energy (Bystrom et al., 2019).

Human Capabilities and Nature-Based Interventions

Nature-based interventions for people with and without disabilities are also supported by research relating to human potential and capabilities. While different cultures may express human potentials and capabilities differently, certain capabilities seem universal. One foundational capability is the "capability to develop." This capability defines, in part, what it means to be human (Chawla, 2015). Other capabilities—sometimes referred to as the "ten central capabilities"—also seem to be universal and essential for human flourishing. One of the ten central capabilities focuses on "being able to live with the full range of creatures and plants that inhabit the world around us" and "being able to enjoy nature and appreciate its beauty" (Nussbaum, 2011). This capability obviously involves connectedness to nature. Other research, too, links nature connectedness to the promotion of different domains of human well-being (Ward Thompson & Aspinall, 2011).

A recent review of the literature sought to determine if nature connectedness is a basic human psychological need (Baxter & Pelletier, 2018). This review investigated two categories of psychological need: "needs as requirements" and "needs as motives." "Needs as requirements" refer to psychological needs which must be met for a human being to achieve sufficient levels of well-being and to promote growth. "Needs as motives" refer to "a form of motivation that compels individuals to pursue certain incentives or goals." The overall findings of this review provide strong support for the understanding that nature connectedness is a basic psychological need for humans and that this applies to both "needs as requirements" and "needs as motives." The findings of this review also indicate that nature connectedness has a positive impact on human health and functioning.

Another review of the literature analyzed 25 studies exploring the relationship between connection with nature and two types of well-being: eudaimonic well-being and hedonic well-being (Pritchard et al., 2019).

Eudaimonic well-being generally means "functioning well" or "fulfill-ing one's potential." Eudaimonic well-being is also translated as "human flourishing." Hedonic well-being, on the other hand, is about "feeling well" or "having pleasant feelings." This review found that both types of well-being are positively linked to nature connectedness, particularly in the areas of psychological growth and development.

According to E. O. Wilson, a Harvard University researcher and scientist, humans have an innate affinity for the natural world. Wilson (1984) referred to this affinity as "biophilia" and defined it as "the urge to affiliate with other forms of life." He and his colleagues proposed that biophilia is biologically based and integral to the holistic development of humans (Kellert & Wilson, 1993). Related research supports this claim (Gullone, 2000). In *The Biophilic Effect*, Clemens Arvay (2018b) supports this view and presents biomedical research into nature's healing effects on our bodies, minds, and spirits.

Thus, we have scientific evidence that nature is something that we all need, and that biophilia is something we all have. We also learn from research that frequent and meaningful engagement with nature can promote human health and well-being. Research, then, provides strong support for the Bittersweet model. The stories of adults who live at Bittersweet Farms also tell us that the Bittersweet model allows them to experience a rich and rewarding quality of life. Some of these stories are included in this book.

Overview of the Book

The story of Bittersweet Farms is the story of families and caring profes-sionals who were concerned about the future of a group of high school students with ASD who would soon be graduating. At the time, there were no community-based residential or work-related programs which could accommodate their specific disabilities and their unique gifts. The history of Bittersweet Farms and the vision of its founder, Bettye Ruth Kay, are provided in Chapter 1.

This book was motivated in part by the dynamic and ever-concerned parents on the board of directors of Bittersweet Farms. Since its founding, these parents have played an important role in maintaining the focus of the organization and on maintaining the quality of the farm's humanistic ther-apeutic approach. Over the years, parents have seen their adult children transformed by their experience of being part of the Bittersweet commu-nity. They realized that the Bittersweet approach is unique and effective.

In 1983, the first residents were enrolled in the Bittersweet program. The program is still staffed by many of the original professionals who worked with Bettye Ruth Kay. Parents are concerned that once the original staff members retire, new staff will need to be trained in the

Bittersweet model which has proven effective in helping their adult children experience a high quality of life. While the Bittersweet model has always focused on the unique needs and capabilities of individuals with ASD, the model has evolved and has been refined over the years. It has not, however, been formalized in any written form. This book outlines the major components of the original Bittersweet model and current modifications and can be used as a guide in training others in this unique approach to providing services for adults with ASD.

Included in this book are stories about individuals who moved to Bittersweet Farms as young adults and who, over the years, enjoyed a high quality of life made possible through specific interventions designed to meet their unique needs and foster their individual capabilities. A program evaluation profiled 20 residents who have been living at Bittersweet for over 30 years. A quality-of-life scale developed for this population was used to measure improvements in eight domains over time. The results of the program evaluation focusing on the outcomes of the Bittersweet model are presented and discussed in Chapter 8 of this book.

Together, the residents' stories, the program evaluation findings, and a strong theoretical framework attest to the effectiveness of the Bittersweet model. This book was written to help others appreciate the value of this model in providing opportunities for adults with ASD to experience quality of life in a community where their individual strengths and special interests are recognized.

References

Ambler, P. G., Eidels, A., & Gregory, C. (2015). Anxiety and aggression in adolescents with autism spectrum disorders attending mainstream schools. *Research in Autism Spectrum Disorders, 18*, 97–109.

Armstrong, T. (2017). The healing balm of nature: Understanding and supporting the naturalist intelligence in individuals diagnosed with ASD. *Physics of Life Reviews, 20*, 109–111.

Arvay, C. G. (2018a). *The healing code of nature.* Boulder, CO: Sounds True.

Arvay, C. G. (2018b). *The biophilic effect.* Boulder, CO: Sounds True.

Barakat, H. A., Bakr, A., & Zeyad El-Sayad, Z. (2019). Nature as a healer for autistic children. *Alexandria Engineering Journal, 58*(1), 353–366.

Baxter, D. E., & Pelletier, L. G. (2018). Is nature relatedness a basic human psychological need? A critical examination of the extant literature. *Canadian Psychology, 60*(1), 21–34.

Bratman, G. N., Anderson, C. B., Berman, M. G., Cochran, B., de Vries, S., Flanders, J., … Daily, G. C. (2019). Nature and mental health: An ecosystem service perspective. *Science Advances, 5*(7), 1–14.

Bratman, G. N., Daily, G. C., Levy, B. J., & Gross, J. J. (2015). The benefits of nature experience: Improved affect and cognition. *Landscape and Urban Planning, 138*, 41–50.

Bystrom, K., Grahn, P., & Hägerhäll, C. (2019). Vitality from experiences in nature and contact with animals—A way to develop joint attention and social engagement in children with autism? *International Journal of Environmental Research and Public Health, 16*(23), 1–36.

Cassidy, S., Bradley, P., Robinson, J., Allison, C., McHugh, M., & Baron-Cohen, S. (2014). Suicidal ideation and suicide plans or attempts in adults with Asperger's syndrome attending a specialist diagnostic clinic: A clinical cohort study. *Lancet, 1*(2), 142–147.

Chawla, L. (2015). Benefits of nature contact for children. *Journal of Planning Literature, 30*(4), 433–452.

DaWalt, L. S., Usher, L. V., Greenberg, J. S., & Mailick, M. R. (2019). Friendships and social participation as markers of quality of life of adolescents and adults with fragile X syndrome and autism. *Autism, 23*(3), 383–393.

Gullone, E. (2000). The biophilia hypothesis and life in the 21st century: Increasing mental health or increasing pathology? *Journal of Happiness Studies, 1*(3), 293–321.

Hirvikoski, T., & Blomqvist, M. (2015). High self-perceived stress and poor coping in intellectually able adults with autism spectrum disorder. *Autism, 19*(6), 752–757.

Hong, J., Bishop-Fitzpatrick, L., Smith, L. E., Greenberg, J. S., & Mailick, M. R. (2016). Factors associated with subjective quality of life of adults with autism spectrum disorder: Self-report versus maternal reports. *Journal of Autism and Developmental Disorders, 46*(4), 1368–1378.

Howlin, P. (2000). Outcome in adult life for more able individuals with autism or asperger syndrome. *Women's Health, 4*(1), 183–194.

Kellert, S. R., & Wilson, E. O. (1993). *The biophilia hypothesis*. Washington, DC: Island Press.

Khanna, R., Jariwala-Parikh, K., West-Strum, D., & Mahabaleshwarkar, R. (2014). Health-related quality of life and its determinants among adults with autism. *Research in Autism Spectrum Disorders, 8*(3), 157–167.

Kuo, M. (2015). How might contact with nature promote human health? Promising mechanisms and a possible central pathway. *Frontiers in Psychology, 6*, 1093. https://doi.org/10.3389/fpsyg.2015.01093

Lever, A. G., & Geurts, H. H. (2016). Psychiatric co-occurring symptoms and disorders in young, middle-aged, and older adults with autism spectrum disorder. *Journal of Autism and Developmental Disorders, 46*(6), 1916–1930.

Li, D., Larsen, L., Yang, Y., Wang, L., Zhai, Y., & Sullivan, W. C. (2019). Exposure to nature for children with autism spectrum disorder: Benefits, caveats, and barriers. *Health and Place, 55*, 71–79.

Lidstone, P., Uljarević, M., Sullivan, J., Rodgers, J., McConachie, H., Freeston, M., … Leekam, S. (2014). Relations among restricted and repetitive behaviors, anxiety and sensory features in children with autism spectrum disorders. *Research in Autism Spectrum Disorders, 8*(2), 82–92.

Marriage, S., Wolverton, A., & Marriage, K. (2009). Autism spectrum disorder grown up: A chart review of adult functioning. *Journal of the Canadian Academy of Child and Adolescent Psychiatry, 18*(4), 322–328.

Mason, D., McConachie, H., Garland, G., Petrou, A., Rodgers, J., & Parr, J. R. (2018). Predictors of quality of life for autistic adults. *Autism Research, 11*(8), 1138–1147.

Masterton, W., Carver, H., Parks, T., & Park, K. (2020). Greenspace interventions for mental health in clinical and non-clinical populations: What works, for whom, and in what circumstances? *Health and Place, 64*, 1–19.

Mesibov, G. B., Shea, V., & Schopler, E. (2004). *The TEACCH approach to autism spectrum disorders*. New York: Springer.

Moss, P., Mandy, W., & Howlin, P. (2017). Child and adult factors related to quality of life in adults with autism. *Journal of Autism and Developmental Disorders, 47*(6), 1830–1837.

Nussbaum, M. C. (2011). Human capabilities and animal lives: Conflict, wonder, law: A symposium. *Journal of Human Development, 18*(3), 317–321.

Pritchard, A., Richardson, M., Sheffield, D., & McEwan, K. (2019). The relationship between nature connectedness and eudaimonic well-being: A meta-analysis. *Journal of Happiness Studies, 21*(3), 1145–1167.

Rentry, J., & Roeyers, H. (2006). Quality of life in high-functioning adults with autism spectrum disorder. *Autism, 10*(5), 511–524.

Reyes-Riveros, R., Altamirano, A., Barrera, F. D. L., Rozas-Vasquez, D., Vieli, L., & Meli, P. (2021). Linking public urban green spaces and human well-being: A systematic review. *Urban Forestry and Urban Greening, 61,* 127105. https://doi.org/10.1016/j.ufug.2021.127105

Robertson, S. M. (2010). Neurodiversity, quality of life, and autistic adults: Shifting research and professional focuses onto real-life challenges. *Disability Studies Quarterly, 30*(1), 27.

Schalock, R. L. (2004). The concept of quality of life: What we know and do not know. *Journal of Intellectual Disability Research, 48*(3), 203–216.

Simonoff, E., Pickles, A., Charman, T., Chandler, S., Loucas, T., & Baird, G. (2008). Psychiatric disorders in children with autism spectrum disorders: Prevalence, comorbidity, and associated factors in a population-derived sample. *Journal of the American Academy of Child and Adolescent Psychiatry, 47*(8), 921–929.

Steinhausen, H. C., Mohr Jensen, C., & Lauritsen, M. (2016). A systematic review and meta-analysis of the long-term overall outcome of autism spectrum disorders in adolescence and adulthood. *Acta Psychiatrica Scandinavica, 133*(6), 445–452.

Twohig-Bennett, C., & Jones, A. (2018). The health benefits of the great outdoors: A systematic review and meta-analysis of greenspace exposure and healthy outcomes. *Environmental Research, 166*, 628–637.

Ulrich, R. S. (1983). Aesthetic and affective response to natural environment. In I. Altman & J. F. Wohlwill (Eds.), *Behavior and the natural environment* (pp. 85–125). New York: Springer.

Ward-Thompson, C., & Aspinall, P. (2011). Natural environments and their impact on activity, health, and quality of life. *Applied Psychology: Health and Well-Being, 3*(3), 230–260.

White, K., Flanagan, T. D., & Nadig, A. (2018). Examining the relationship between self-determination and quality of life in young adults with autism spectrum disorder. *Journal of Developmental and Physical Disabilities, 30*(6), 735–754.

Wilson, E. O. (1984). *Biophilia: The human bond with other species*. Cambridge, MA: Harvard University Press.

1 History and Vision of Bittersweet Farms

This Is Bittersweet …

… a therapeutic community for adults with autism founded on an understanding that learning and growth are lifelong processes. The Bittersweet community involves an interdisciplinary team including the partnership of participants, parents, staff, medical personnel, therapists, and other service providers. The program, organization, and environment offer endless opportunities for continuing growth and learning (Figure 1.1).

The Roots of Bittersweet

The idea of Bittersweet Farms took root in 1973, the year the first public school in Toledo, Ohio, offered a class for children and adolescents with autism spectrum disorder (ASD). Bettye Ruth Kay taught this class of students. At that time, students with special needs were typically assigned to segregated classrooms where the emphasis was on "improving" a deficit skill or "eliminating" an undesirable behavior. For example, in an effort to improve fine motor control and eye–hand coordination, a student would be given a task stacking blocks. When successfully completed, he or she would be given smaller blocks to stack. Many children, including those with disabilities other than autism, can be taught in this way. However, because of the unique neurological condition inherent in autism, learning through sequential tasking does not usually work.

Bettye Ruth was aware that most students with ASD were considered incapable of learning socially appropriate behaviors and skills. She surmised, however, that the lack of student progress had to do with the absence of motivation. One characteristic of autism is the tendency to engage in non-functional rather than purposeful activities. People with autism tend to focus on individual details and have difficulty understanding how things relate to each other. They also have difficulty imagining

DOI: 10.4324/9781003271048-2

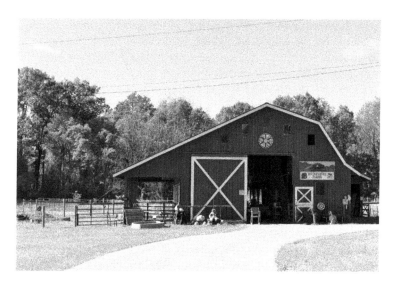

Figure 1.1 Bittersweet Residents and Staff Work in Partnership in Purposeful Jobs Doing the Hard Work of Caring for Farm Animals.

the possible outcomes of their actions. In her assigned basement room in a Toledo, Ohio high school, Bettye Ruth incorporated woodworking and crafts as central components of her teaching. The process of creating something concrete and meaningful became a focus of the student's day. Therapeutic goals were built into individual student efforts. The purposeful activity also played a pivotal role in promoting positive interactions and communication among her students.

At the same time, Bettye Ruth grew increasingly aware of the isolation and lack of services for people with autism. She knew that all humans have a craving to belong and for the interdependence that is part of a community. Her students were no different. However, most services and programs available for this population focused on managing the challenging behaviors rather than promoting staff and participants working together with mutual assistance and cooperation to develop a sense of belonging for everyone.

As Bettye Ruth was developing her treatment approaches, parents of these students were expressing anxiety as to their children's future. As adults, where would their children live? What kind of supports would be available? Would his or her functioning improve, stay the same, or deteriorate? Most importantly, what quality of life would they experience?

The families of these young people had cause for concern. Adult services for those with autism were scarce and most often inappropriate. Although the Individuals with Disabilities Education Act (IDEA) ensures that all students with autism receive free appropriate public education, no such law ensures free and appropriate services for adults.

Even though families of individuals with autism universally deal with these questions, very little was known about the unfolding life course of people with autism. Almost all of the literature on families focused on early childhood and school-age children (Seltzer et al., 2001).

Bettye Ruth started meeting regularly with the parents. She relentlessly pursued research and sought out experts to assist in designing a blueprint for the future of her students. What she most wanted for them was a setting that would promote interaction and community, address behavior management concerns, and provide opportunities for continuing learning and development. What Bettye Ruth wanted for her students was a program specially tailored to meet their unique needs. She wanted her students to have an opportunity to achieve their highest potential and experience a rich quality of life.

Finding a Model

One program, Somerset Court in Great Britain, caught Bettye Ruth's attention. She arranged to visit Somerset Court where she observed residents actively engaged in a variety of tasks in the farm-like environment provided. Such tasks included weaving, groundskeeping, carpentry, knitting, and home maintenance. These tasks—along with self-care activities—promoted a sense of dignity, independence, and pride. Bettye Ruth noted how these positive outcomes fostered a feeling of community and respect among the residents and staff (Elgar, 1999).

Bettye Ruth realized that a farmstead model would provide a setting that encouraged interaction, communication, and positive relationships among the participants and staff—all key components of quality of life. The wide variety of purposeful activities on a farm would be motivating and result in completed projects, which would then promote self-worth and self-esteem. A large farm encourages physical activity during work hours and provides a setting for endless opportunities for physical recreation, such as hiking and biking. Physical activity, in addition to reducing anxiety and stress, also promotes an overall sense of well-being.

The variety of activities on a farm would also allow participants to have choices of activities, something other settings generally cannot provide. The opportunity to make independent choices would give participants a chance to do what they like to do and engage in activities that match their interests and gifts. It would also allow participants to move at their own pace while engaged in meaningful activities. Bettye Ruth found the idea of a farm setting which promoted self-determination, social inclusion, and interdependence with the staff and the rural community appealing. After visiting Somerset Court, she resolved to develop a program based on this model for adults with autism. This resolve proved to be a catalyst for the development of a special Northwest Ohio community for adults with autism: Bittersweet Farms.

From Dream to Reality

Thus began the arduous task of creating a concrete proposal for a farmstead based on Bettye Ruth's vision of what that could be. She, along with parents, enlisted the support of key community members and legislators who would be instrumental in making the dream become a reality. It was a daunting task. The fiscal support needed to develop and maintain the program was immense. Locating a site for the farmstead presented many challenges for the planners. Bettye Ruth and her cadre of parents and supporters persevered. Finally, an 80-acre farm located southwest of Toledo, Ohio, was purchased. A grant of $457,365.00 from the Ohio Department of Mental Retardation provided funds for land acquisition and to build a residence for 15 adults with ASD. In 1983, the first residents were enrolled at Bittersweet Farms, the first farmstead community for adults with ASD in North America.

The buildings on Bittersweet Farms include a two-story house for residents and staff, a large barn, several greenhouses, and a woodworking shop. The activities on the farm reflect a belief in both the intrinsic and therapeutic value of meaningful work. All residents at Bittersweet participate in the management and stewardship of the farm. The rationale for a farm-life model for adults with ASD is based, in part, on the way such a model provides purposeful work for every level of ability (Kay, 1990).

Bittersweet is owned and operated by a non-profit organization, the Autistic Community of Northwest Ohio, Inc. The farm was named for the Bittersweet vines found on the property—symbolizing the potential of the Bittersweet program as well as the bittersweet lives of those with autism.

Bettye Ruth's pioneering efforts on behalf of those with autism did not go unnoticed. The US Congress recognized her achievements with a special commendation. She was inducted into the Ohio Women's Hall of Fame for her vision and tireless efforts on behalf of persons with autism, and for making the Bittersweet dream become a reality.

Bittersweet Today

Bittersweet Farms is an example of a community-based non-institutional program providing residential and therapeutic services for adults with ASD. Original activities on the farm focused on self-sufficiency through the cultivation of farm animals and crops. The concept was later expanded to include the creation of products that could be sold commercially. Today, Bittersweet Farms includes a woodworking shop, a ceramics and art studio, and a weaving loom. While residents are actively engaged in meaningful work much of the time, the Bittersweet model also recognizes the importance of recreation and leisure. Because people with ASD generally have trouble organizing their free time purposefully, physical and social supports are carefully planned to help residents enjoy a wide range of recreation and leisure activities. Opportunities for physically active recreation include running, hiking, and biking, all of which provide sensory input for residents who have sensory processing deficits. Social activities include a variety of indoor and outdoor games and participation in special interest clubs, such as handbell choir.

Community integration through work and recreation has always been a focus of Bittersweet Farms. A number of approaches are used to promote this integration. Bittersweet sells its creative products through the local marketplace and provides frequent outings and trips into the community. Bittersweet Farms has also initiated a "reverse" integration program where community members are invited to the farm. One such program, called "Fall on the Farm," brings community members to the farm where they can participate in tours and hayrides and watch demonstrations in the vocational workshops.

Core Values

Autism does not define who an individual is. Rather it is a descriptor of characteristics common to a disability. It is those characteristics—specifically those related to behaviors—which are often the focus of intervention programs or treatment. The perception that some people are "normal" and others are deficient and need to be repaired in some way is still a part of a society that values uniformity. Lost in this approach is the human individuality so integral to the celebrated diversity and accomplishments of our civilization. Bettye Ruth acknowledged this individualism as a cornerstone of the Bittersweet program and community. She emphasized the contributions and value of each individual, both staff and resident, as essential components for building an integrated program. The resulting teamwork created a real community of purpose: "The Bettye Ruth Way."

The Bittersweet model is designed to address the needs and promote the growth of adults with ASD in every area of life. The focus of this approach is on quality of life. Understanding and appreciating people with ASD are fundamental to the entire process. The physical venue is a farm; the social venue an extended family community. For the residents, staff, day participants, and visitors, Bittersweet Farms is

> a relaxed, friendly, beautiful place to live and work where life is enjoyable and meaningful. There is a sense of wholeness about everything, from the concern for all aspects of the individual's life to a harmony with the environment and with nature.
>
> (Kay, 1990, p. 320)

Community, closeness to nature, quality of life, purpose, and respect for individualism—these are core values of the Bittersweet model. These core values are reflected in the way people at Bittersweet spend their days caring for the land and its products, for the animals living on the farm, and for each other.

References

Elgar, S. (1999). Treatment settings in the United Kingdom for autistic adults. In N. S. Giddan & J. J. Giddan (Eds.), *Autistic adults in bittersweet farms* (pp. 67–75). Binghamton, NY: The Haworth Press.

Kay, B. R. (1990). Bittersweet farms. *Journal of Autism and Developmental Disorders*, *20*(3), 309–321.

Seltzer, N. M., Krauss, M. W., Orsmond, G. I., & Vestal, C. (2001). Families of adolescents and adults with autism: Uncharted territory. *International Review of Research in Mental Retardation, 23*, 267–294.

2 The Bittersweet Model

From Theory to Practice

The seeds of Bittersweet have their origin in two philosophical approaches that guide all aspects of program planning and implementation. First, there is an understanding and appreciation of the diversity apparent in all humankind. This is embodied in the work of Dr Howard Gardner's critically acclaimed theory of multiple intelligences (Gardner, 1983). The core of the program, though, reflects the thoughts and research of Abraham Maslow's Hierarchy of Needs (Maslow, 1954). It is the adaptation of Maslow's theory that provides the foundation for program planning, implementation, evaluation, and staff training. The Bittersweet model also reflects an understanding of the benefits of engagement with nature for human development and well-being, especially for people with autism spectrum disorder (ASD).

Multiple Intelligences

The results of IQ tests, achievement exams, and report card grades are traditionally used as indicators of one's capabilities. Data from such quantifiers provide an appraisal of what we typically consider intelligence—the linguistic and logical-mathematical aptitudes valued by mainstream culture.

In the early 1980s, Dr Howard Gardner, a professor at Harvard, suggested that this understanding of "intelligence" is too limited. He proposed eight different intelligences to include a broader range of human potential (Gardner, 1983).

Dr Gardner (1983) hypothesized that individuals show gifts in intelligences beyond linguistic and mathematical. He observed that IQ results as predictors of individual potential ignore the special aptitudes of many people. For example, athletes, whose kinesthetic ability enables them to hit a ball traveling at 90 plus miles per hour,

DOI: 10.4324/9781003271048-3

Table 2.1 Multiple Intelligences

Dr. Gardner's Eight Different Intelligences	
Intelligence	Definition
1. Linguistic-Verbal	Word Smart
2. Logical-Mathematical	Number/Reasoning Smart
3. Spatial	Picture Smart
4. Bodily-Kinesthetic	Body Smart
5. Musical	Music Smart
6. Interpersonal	People Smart
7. Intrapersonal	Self Smart
8. Naturalist	Nature Smart

artists who envision and create impressive photographs and paintings, counselors with insights into human behaviors, builders, musicians, designers, environmentalists, and entrepreneurs—all enrich the world in which we live. Dr Gardner's work calls attention to the multiplicity of intelligences humans exhibit.

Most residents and day students come to Bittersweet with thick folders of reports specifying all types of clinical findings, observations, and client background. While this information is important, few of these records provide clues as to the special attributes the individual may possess. If there is a special talent, it's usually classified as an anomaly. If the individual demonstrates an extraordinary skill, such as playing the piano or the ability to calculate difficult mathematical problems ("Rain Man"), he or she may be given another misunderstood label: that of a savant.

According to Gardner, everyone has each type of intelligence to varying degrees, but culture and experience influence the development of a particular type of intelligence. Each intelligence needs a related stimulating physical and social environment to maximize its development. As the following examples illustrate, life at Bittersweet Farms provides residents with many opportunities to thrive in their own unique ways.

Valuing Diversity: The Bittersweet Way

Seeking out the special aptitudes of the residents is a key component of the Bittersweet program. Staff members embrace the notion that each person has gifts and interests to share.

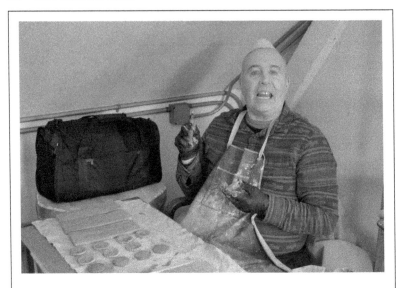

Figure 2.1 This Resident has Exceptional Fine Motor Skills and an Interest in Handling Very Small Items. He Finds Joy in Working with Clay.

One of the women with ASD is amazingly knowledgeable about vegetable crops. Her knowledge and skills are used in a meaningful way by involving her in developing planting guides for the gardens at Bittersweet. Some residents receive training and support to develop special skills. One resident, for example, expressed a keen interest in machinery and keys. She went through the necessary training and can now work as a locksmith. Another resident displayed a passion for baking. With support, he was able to start his own micro business, baking specialty pies.

The participants at Bittersweet have a multiplicity of intelligences and gifts that enrich the community. Some of the residents create works of art that are sold in the storefront on the farm or are shown at art exhibits in the community. Residents interested in horticulture help produce the food, which is not only served at Bittersweet, but also sold at farmers' markets. Basil is one example of a food grown and processed on the farm to be distributed to local stores. Residents interested in the process use the basil for making pesto, which is popular in the local market. Residents with a talent for woodworking make furniture and small wooden items that are sold at local festivals. Some residents with athletic talents compete in regional and national sports competitions. Their achievements and the medals they win contribute to community pride. As these examples illustrate, the special gifts and talents promoted through the Bittersweet model help to create an interdependent and enriching community.

Hierarchy of Needs

American psychologist Abraham Maslow developed the theory of human motivation known as Maslow's Hierarchy of Needs (1954). Unlike most psychologists who studied negative human behavior, Maslow sought out the good in people; "the best of humanity." He chose to focus on human potential, believing that all humans strive to reach their highest levels of capability. Maslow's Hierarchy of Needs is usually presented in the shape of a pyramid or triangle, with self-actualization at the peak. According to Maslow, this hierarchy of needs is common to all people.

Maslow (1954) proposed five categories of needs. In hierarchical order, these are physiological, safety, love, esteem, and self-actualization. Maslow believed that needs lower in the hierarchy must be satisfied before individuals can attend to higher-level needs. According to this theory, higher-level needs begin to emerge only when an individual recognizes that his or her lower-level needs have been satisfied.

The five levels of need identified by Maslow, represented as a pyramid (Figure 2.2), include

1. Biological and physiological. These are the most basic needs for survival: air to breathe, water to drink, food to eat, shelter, warmth, etc.

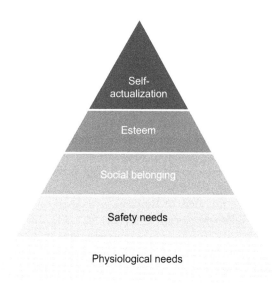

Figure 2.2 Maslow's Hierarchy of Needs Triangle Divided into Five Sections with Each Section Labeled According to Maslow's Hierarchy of Needs.

2. Safety. Once physiological needs have been met, individuals seek safety and security. They develop a need for structure, some limits, stability, freedom from danger, and absence of threat. They may not be concerned about hunger and thirst but have fears and anxieties about safety.

3. Belongingness and love. A prerequisite human need for achieving a sense of self-worth is to belong and be loved. A sense of belonging depends on an appreciation and acceptance of diversity. Families, friendships, and community are priorities at this level of need.

4. Esteem. Self-esteem can be met through mastery or achievement in a given area or through gaining respect or recognition from others. Self-esteem or self-respect depends on feeling competent and confident in one's own capabilities. Maslow stressed that only when we are "anchored in community" do we develop the self-esteem needed to assure ourselves of our own individual worth.

5. Self-actualization. Finally, when one achieves a sense of self-worth, he or she is free to pursue his or her own unique gifts and talents.

Maslow maintained that individuals do not seek the satisfaction of a need at one level until the previous "level of need" has been met. The most basic need is for physiological survival: shelter, warmth, food, drink, etc. Once these requirements have been met, the individual is able to address the need for safety and security, including freedom from danger and the absence of threat. Then belonging, or love—usually found in families, friendships, and within community —becomes the priority. Only when "anchored in community" can one achieve self-esteem and be assured of one's own self-worth. Self-esteem can be met through mastery or achievement in a given field or endeavor and by the recognition of others. Self-esteem enables freedom to pursue one's own self-actualization.

Maslow viewed all these needs as essentially survival needs. Even love and esteem are needed for the maintenance of health. According to Maslow, we all have these needs "built into us genetically, like instincts." Maslow's humanist views are basic to the approach used at Bittersweet— the right to be human.

The first concern of the founders of Bittersweet focused on finding a setting where young adults with autism could live in a safe and structured environment. This concern was consistent with Maslow's theory about the fundamental need for survival, which includes a safe place to live. The 80-acre farm provides such a setting. The farm, located in a rural community, offers a calm setting with protections from the stresses of a fast-paced society that often does not understand the unique needs of adults with ASD. The farm setting also offers a variety of meaningful and interesting activities, which allow participation at differing levels of ability. While many people with ASD can adapt well in more typical settings, the participants of the Bittersweet program have greater challenges than others and were not successful living and working at home. The farmstead provides a safe, structured environment with opportunities to interact with the larger agricultural community during structured activities.

Many of the residents, if placed in other settings, would face critical safety concerns. Some adults with ASD tend to wander and may get lost in neighborhoods. They may also be unaware of traffic-related dangers and have problems with law enforcement procedures. They may become agitated if police are not highly trained to recognize that they have behavior challenges or do not know how to intervene appropriately. People with ASD can also be taken advantage of financially and sexually. The farmstead model is designed to meet the residents' need for protection, security, order, and stability—needs outlined in the second level of Maslow's hierarchy,

The third level of Maslow's hierarchy is belongingness and love. At Bittersweet, that level of human need is addressed through a partnership approach. Staff members do not supervise participants while they work, but are partners with them in all activities. For example, horticulturists work side by side with participants planting crops and harvesting. This partnership approach encourages social interaction which people with ASD want but have very few skills to achieve. Staff members become friends, and a sense of community is developed. One participant refers to the Bittersweet community as her family. She loves spending vacation time and holidays there where she feels the warmth of the staff and the friendship of the other participants.

The fourth and fifth levels of Maslow's hierarchy, esteem and self-actualization, are addressed through the vocational program at Bittersweet, where participants are free to choose the work they most enjoy and which allows their gifts and talents to be utilized and appreciated. The Bittersweet model is based on the understanding that self-esteem develops in a loving and supportive community in which members of that community appreciate the work and talents of each other. Self-actualization—or becoming what you are capable of becoming—implies individualization, which is the basis of Bittersweet programming. The goal for each resident is to achieve the personal growth and fulfillment that spring from a feeling of self-worth and belonging.

The Maslow hierarchy provides a theoretical basis for the Bittersweet program; yet, it is the *adaptations* of the hierarchy that make the approach successful for Bittersweet residents. Maslow described the process toward self-actualization in hierarchical terms. The theory implies that each step must be achieved before moving on to the next. Although this framework may be useful for analyzing behaviors and planning individual programs for individuals without autism, there is an inherent need for flexibility when working with adults with ASD. The neurological characteristics that define autism are distinct. For people with ASD, changes in behavior, situations, and needs occur without predictability. "Progress" achieved in the past may disappear without warning. Movement toward a given goal may stall or change depending on many variables.

Like Maslow's hierarchy, the Bittersweet model provides the framework for participants' journey toward self-actualization and a higher quality of life. Yet, for people with ASD, different components of the model must be continually revisited and revised as participants' needs change.

Engagement with Nature

Engagement with nature is something everyone needs for optimal physical, social, and emotional development. This may be especially important for people with ASD. Fortunately, all people seem to have an affinity for nature. We call this biophilia. According to Howard Gardner (1983), many people have something else, as well—naturalistic intelligence. This intelligence—sometimes referred to as "nature smart"—includes the ability to recognize plants, animals, and other parts of the natural environment. Naturalistic intelligence also deals with sensing patterns in and making connections with elements in the natural world. As living and working on a farm provide many opportunities for deep engagement with the natural world, Bittersweet Farms offers an environment where naturalistic intelligence can flourish.

Recent research suggests that some of the strengths of individuals with ASD are associated with high naturalist intelligence. These strengths could then be used to create supportive environments for individuals with ASD (Armstrong, 2017; Masataka, 2017). Some research also suggests that, while everyone can benefit from engagement with nature, the benefits of such engagement may be greater for individuals with ASD (Barakat, 2019). Such benefits include improved communication, more positive social interactions, increased physical activity, cognitive development, and greater emotional affect (Armstrong, 2017). The literature on the nature benefits for people with ASD includes such phrases as "nature as a healer" (Barakat, 2019) and "the healing balm of nature" (Armstrong, 2017). Nature, then, in addition to the other benefits it offers, can be a source of solace for people with ASD.

Recognizing naturalistic intelligence in people with ASD calls attention to the provocative concept of neurodiversity—the idea that certain developmental disabilities, including autism, aren't inherently pathological but are, instead, natural human variations (Masataka, 2017; Robertson, 2010; Silberman, 2017). The concept of neurodiversity was first introduced in the late 1990s, when it was initially referred to as "neurological pluralism." Researchers and others were soon relating the concept of neurodiversity to biodiversity, which suggests that natural variations in the world of nature make it healthier and more resilient. In 1998, Harvey Blume, a writer for *The Atlantic*, made the term popular by stating that "Neurodiversity may be every bit as crucial for the human race as biodiversity is for life in general" (Blume, 1998).

The term "neurodiversity" refers to the variation in neurocognitive functioning within humans. Neurodiversity is a fact, not a perspective or idea. A related term, "neurotypical," refers to a style of neurocognitive functioning that is viewed as "normal" within dominant social standards. Autism is one form of neurodivergence (Robertson, 2010).

Research on neurodiversity challenges the deficiency-oriented approach often used in work related to people with ASD. Neurodiversity calls attention to the strengths and gifts versus the "disabilities" of people with ASD. Such gifts include enhanced auditory and visual discrimination capabilities, which often manifest as hyper-sensation and hyper-attention to detail. These abilities, which are highly adaptive for living in nature, suggest that during prehistoric times, these abilities may have had an evolutionary advantage (Armstrong, 2017). The characteristics of ASD, then, "are not an error of nature but an invaluable part of human genetic variability" (Masataka, 2017: 104). People with ASD may seem disabled because their gifts are not in sync with modern civilization. Simple forms of exposure to nature could possibly ameliorate some of the related concerns and improve their quality of life (Matasaka, 2017).

Other research conducted over the past several decades supports the many benefits of nature for humans. One comprehensive review shows that people with more frequent and intense engagement with nature tend to be happier, healthier, and more creative than people who spend little time engaged with nature (Hartig, 2014). One interesting finding of this review relates to how being active in natural settings may yield health benefits over and above the benefits of physical activity in other environments. The beneficial effects of "green exercise" relate to positive moods, self-esteem, enjoyment, and motivation (Matasaka, 2017).

Another comprehensive review of the literature found 44 examples of positive associations between green space and prosocial behavior. The positive behavioral outcomes identified included offering help, sharing, cooperating, and comforting (Putra et al., 2020).

Further research by a multidisciplinary team of health-related professionals identified a list of 20 evidence-based health benefits of nature contact. The team based their work on a broad definition of health to include physical and mental health, social well-being, academic and job performance, and happiness (Frumkin et al., 2017). Of the 20 benefits, a number of them—such as reduced depression and anxiety, greater happiness and life satisfaction, reduced aggression, and increased social connectedness—may have special relevance for adults with ASD.

Anxiety and lack of stress management skills are concerns for many people with ASD. Some reasons for increased anxiety in people with ASD include difficulties in understanding social situations and expectations, social communication difficulties, sensory issues, and changes in routines. Anxiety and stress aren't "stand-alone" problems. They overflow into physical and mental health issues. Research on stress shows that persistent stress—often experienced by people with ASD—can lead to permanent damage to the human brain (Arvay, 2018a).

The fact that mental illness tends to be more common in people on the autism spectrum than in the general population, could be due to the increased stress and anxiety they experience in their daily lives. Environmental psychologists have found that "being away" can alleviate the experience of stress. "Being away" places a distance between social burdens and concerns. Engagement with nature tends to provide a "being away" experience for many people (Arvay, 2018a).

Restorative Benefits of Nature

Two established theoretical frameworks also support the idea that people with ASD may benefit from spending time in nature. Both of these theories relate to the restorative benefits of nature. One theory, the Stress Reduction Theory (SRT), suggests that nature reduces stress. This theory is based on the idea that viewing vegetation and other natural-appearing environmental features can evoke positive emotions that block negative thoughts and emotions (Bratman et al., 2015). The other theory, the Attention Restoration Theory (ART), suggests that nature can replenish or restore one's capacity for directed attention. This theory is based on the understanding that features of the natural environment attract and hold a person's attention without effort. This form of attention—referred to as "fascination"—allows the neurocognitive mechanism involved in effortful directed attention to rest (Markevych et al., 2017).

Many of our daily living activities—working, interacting with others, self-care activities—require directed attention. This form of attention costs us energy and can lead to fatigue and stress. Fascination—the other form of attention—doesn't cost us any energy or exertion. It can, in fact, regenerate mental energy (Arvay, 2018a). Because nature is full of elements that fascinate us or attract our attention effortlessly, engagement with nature can help us recover our capacity for directed attention.

As people with ASD tend to experience high levels of attention difficulties and stress-related concerns, the restorative powers of nature may be especially helpful for them. Both SRT and ART are supported by a rich body of research (Bratman et al., 2015; Kaplan & Kaplan, 1989; Ulrich, 1981; Ulrich et al., 1991).

Engagement with Animals

Engagement with animals also seems to have special benefits for people with ASD. This may be due, in part, to the fact that animals (especially pets) are a source of non-judgmental and positive affection (Matasaka, 2017). The presence of animals can reduce loneliness and may serve as "distractors" for individuals when faced with stressful situations. Of special relevance for people with ASD, engagement with animals and other forms of nature tends to decrease anxiety and buffer stress.

Engagement with animals can also promote the social skills of people with ASD. One study showed that children with ASD demonstrated more social approach behaviors (such as talking, looking at faces, and making tactile contact) in the presence of animals compared to toys. The children in this study also displayed more prosocial behaviors and positive affect (such as smiling and laughing) as well as less self-focused behaviors and negative affect (i.e., frowning, crying, and whining) in the presence of animals compared to toys (O'Haire et al., 2013). While this study was conducted with children, the benefits of animal-assisted therapies apply to people of all ages (Louv, 2006).

Some research has focused specifically on the benefits of farm animals for people with mental health concerns. According to Arvay (2018a), contact with farm animals can promote clearly measurable psychotherapeutic effects in people with mental illness. He notes how farm animals—goats, sheep, horses, cattle, pigs, and so on—"are social animals with distinct personalities and are useful for therapeutic interaction with people" (p. 129). Arvay discusses how regular involvement with and nurturing of farm animals can lead to decreased depressive symptoms and increased ability for coping with problems.

Quality of Life Considerations

Honoring the neurodiverse abilities of adults with ASD and providing environments where their strengths can be maximized and their weaknesses minimized contribute to their quality of life (Armstrong, 2017). "Greening" the environments in which people with ASD live and work is one way to engage their naturalist proclivities and contribute to their quality of life (Masataka, 2017).

The physical and social environment of Bittersweet Farms is one in which the human needs of the residents are recognized and their special interests and gifts encouraged. Bittersweet Farms is more than a place; it's a community of belonging and purpose. Such a community values the individuality of each person and promotes the quality of life for all involved.

References

Armstrong, T. (2017). The healing balm of nature: Understanding and supporting the naturalist intelligence in individuals diagnosed with ASD. *Physics of Life Reviews, 20,* 109–111.

Arvay, C. G. (2018a). *The healing code of nature.* Boulder, CO: Sounds True.

Barakat, H. A., Bakr, A., & Zeyad El-Sayad, Z. (2019). Nature as a healer for autistic children. *Alexandria Engineering Journal, 58*(1), 353–366.

Blume, H. (1998, September). On the neurological underpinnings of geekdom. *The Atlantic.* https://www.theatlantic.com/magazine/archive/1998/09/neurodiversity/305909/

Bratman, G. N., Daily, G. C., Levy, B. J., & Gross, J. J. (2015). The benefits of nature experience: Improved affect and cognition. *Landscape and Urban Planning, 138,* 41–50.

Frumkin, H., Bratman, G. N., Breslow, S. J., Cockran, B., Kahn, P. H., Lawler, J. J., … Wood, S. A. (2017). Nature contact and human health: A research agenda. *Environmental Health Perspectives, 125*(7). https://doi.org/10.1289/EHP1663

Gardner, H. (1983). *Frames of mind: The theory of multiple intelligences.* New York: Basic Books.

Hartig, T., Mitchell, R., de Vries, S., & Frumkin, H. (2014). Nature and health. *Annual Review of Public Health, 35,* 207–228.

Kaplan, R., & Kaplan, S. (1989). *The experience of nature: A psychological perspective.* Cambridge: Cambridge University Press.

Louv, R. (2006). *Last child in the woods: Saving our children from nature-deficit disorder.* Chapel Hill, NC: Algonquin.

Markevych, I., Schoierer, J., Hartig, T., Chudnovsky, A., Hystad, P., Dzhambov, A. M., … Feng, X. (2017). Exploring pathways linking greenspace to health: Theoretical and methodological guidance. *Environmental Research, 158,* 301–317.

Masataka, N. (2017). Implications of the idea of neurodiversity for understanding the origins of developmental disorders. *Physics of Life Reviews, 20,* 85–108.

Maslow, A. H. (1954). *Motivation and personality.* New York: Harper & Brothers.

O'Haire, M. E., McKenzie, S. J., Beck, A. M., & Slaughter, V. (2013). Social behaviors increase in children with autism in the presence of animals compared to toys. *PLoS One, 8*(2), e57010. https://doi.org/10.1371/journal.pone.0057010

Putra, I. G. N. E., Astell-Burt, T., Cliff, D. P., Vella, S. A., John, E. E., & Feng, X. (2020). The relationship between green space and prosocial behaviour among children and adolescents: A systematic review. *Frontiers in Psychology, 11.* https://doi.org/10.3389/fpsyg.2020.00859

Robertson, S. M. (2010). Neurodiversity, quality of life, and autistic adults: Shifting research and professional focuses onto real-life challenges. *Disability Studies Quarterly, 30*(1), 27.

Silberman, S. (2017). Beyond "deficit-based" thinking in autism research. *Physics of Life Reviews, 20,* 119–121.

Ulrich, R. S. (1981). Natural versus urban scenes: Some psychophysiological effects. *Environment and Behavior, 13*(5), 523–556.

Ulrich, R., Simons, R., Losito, B., Fiorito, E., Miles, M., & Zelson, M. (1991). Stress recovery during exposure to natural and urban environments. *Journal of Environmental Psychology, 11*(3), 201–230.

3 A Firm Foundation

Structure and Support

Buildings need a solid foundation in order to support them or cracks will soon appear and the walls will collapse. Plants must have a healthy root system if they are to grow and thrive. So it is with the Bittersweet Farms community. Structure is the base upon which the entire program depends. Without structure, the program would collapse.

This chapter presents the rationale for developing a solid structure as a prerequisite for program building. The focus is on routines, individualized schedules, sensory processing considerations, a prosthetic environment, visual and other supports, and strategies for dealing with change. Specific suggestions, along with examples and stories illustrating how to put these structures and supports into practice, are offered. The focus throughout is on creating quality of life for the residents and participants at Bittersweet.

The Importance of Routine and Schedules

Predictable routines—mealtime, bedtime, shopping, getting up and going to school or work—are part of the daily rhythm of our lives. We enjoy these patterns as they provide us with a sense of security and control. When we cannot depend on a routine, or it is unexpectedly disrupted, we lose a sense of control and our behavior often reflects some degree of distress or anxiety. For example, waiting for a connecting flight that is delayed or being "stuck" in traffic on the way to an important appointment may cause many anxious moments. We are uncertain as to how long the delay may last or whether we will arrive at our destination at all. Coping with having no control over the situation and not knowing what will happen next is difficult. In all cases, our sense of well-being is altered. Outcomes may be manifested in physical symptoms and/or emotional behaviors. We yearn for the predictability and structure that routine provides. Although we may feel overwhelmed and out of control

DOI: 10.4324/9781003271048-4

at the time, most of us learn to cope with these everyday occurrences by generalizing past experiences and rationalizing the situation to a manageable level.

For persons with autism the need for structure and routine is critical as their neurological ability to cope with change is limited or missing. Seemingly small variances—some not easy to identify—may create major difficulties for people with autism. Consider the story of Fred, a nonverbal resident at Bittersweet Farms.

COFFEE TIME

Fred exhibited crippling anxiety after finishing a cup of coffee. Staff puzzled over this behavior. Perhaps caffeine was a factor. They noted that if given another cup of coffee the anxiety subsided. They substituted decaffeinated beverages for coffee, but it made no difference. When the drink was finished, the anxiety returned. Thirst did not appear to be a factor.

The problem was resolved after staff developed a visual chart for Fred showing specific times when he would be given certain beverages. Understanding that another beverage would be provided on a set schedule alleviated his distress. Fred's anxiety was rooted in not being confident of when or if he would get another chance for coffee. He needed the communication, structure, and predictability this schedule provided.

Changes in schedules and transitions from one activity and/or setting to another are especially troublesome for many people with autism spectrum disorder (ASD). The slate of what had come to be understood or expected is now wiped clean, and the process of informing, clarifying, and adjusting begins again. When things change, cues from familiar environments or routines are removed causing stress and anxiety. Seemingly minor modifications, such as removing or shifting an item from its given place, can elicit outcomes that seem to be out of proportion to the situation. Reactions vary. Unfortunately, we often respond to these behaviors without identifying their cause.

Routine is essential for people with autism. Some people with ASD have a need to perform ritual behaviors before they feel comfortable with a change or transition taking place. A schedule that makes accommodations for such behaviors can be a source of comfort and contentment.

Some people with ASD may be compelled to carry out an activity to its completion. This makes transition to something else impossible before the task at hand is finished. These self-structuring routines appear to provide a sense of security and comfort. Routines often provide some sense of control to compensate for external disorder. Although these self-structuring behaviors may be viewed as "challenging" or a negative aspect of autism, the need for routine can actually serve as a basis for building positive structure.

Bittersweet has "built in" routine activities that punctuate transitions. From morning breakfast preparation to group teatime before retiring for the night, daily routines are known and expected by the residents. Deviations from these routines may result in problems related to confusion and anxiety. Routines and schedules are anchors in time and space for all of us. But, for people with autism who have difficulties in generalization and rationalization, routines and schedules are essential.

As illustrated in Table 3.1, the general schedule at Bittersweet remains fairly constant from day to day. The vocational habilitation (voc-hab) activities scheduled during the day are individualized to each participant.

Individualized Schedules

Bittersweet participants have varied abilities to complete tasks and to work in vocational settings. Individualized schedules thus become a necessity. Detailed individual schedules are used throughout the Bittersweet programming process. These schedules provide a visual overview of the day's activities. The schedule and each activity on the schedule are carefully planned to provide opportunities for engagement with positive outcomes. For some participants, desired outcomes relate to vocational goals. Related activities often take place in the kitchen or horticultural areas, or involve janitorial tasks. For other participants, prevocational goals are more appropriate. Such goals include improved communication and understanding the nature of a task and its completion. Participants at the prevocational level of functioning may work in some of the same areas as participants at the vocational level of functioning but with different outcome goals. Some of the prevocational activities also occur in the barn and involve groundskeeping tasks.

An individualized schedule is provided to each participant at the beginning of the day. Some participants are able to use their schedules to work independently during all or part of the day. Other participants need time and support to even process the details of their schedules. As the following examples illustrate, Bittersweet staff consider the needs of individual participants as they process their daily schedules. Susan, a

Table 3.1 Typical Weekly Schedule*

TIME	MONDAY	TUESDAY	WEDNESDAY	THURSDAY	FRIDAY	SATURDAY	SUNDAY
7am	Wake up AM care	Wake up AM care	Wake up AM care	Wake up AM care	Wake up AM care	Wake up AM care	Wake up AM care
8am	Breakfast	Breakfast	Breakfast	Breakfast	Breakfast	Breakfast	Breakfast
9am	Voc hab	Voc hab	Voc hab	Voc hab	Voc hab	Breakfast cleanup, morning chores (barn check, compost, etc.)	Breakfast cleanup, morning chores (barn check, compost, etc.)
10am	Voc hab	Voc hab	Voc hab	Voc hab	Voc hab	Hike	Religious experience or hike
11am	Voc hab	Voc hab	Voc hab	Voc hab	Voc hab	Hike	Religious experience or hike
12pm	Lunch	Lunch	Lunch	Lunch	Lunch	Lunch	Lunch
1pm	Voc hab	Voc hab	Voc hab	Voc hab	Voc hab	Hike	Swimming
2pm	Voc hab	Voc hab	Voc hab	Voc hab	Voc hab	Rest & relaxation	Swimming
3pm	Voc hab	Voc hab	Voc hab	Voc hab	Voc hab	Afternoon activity	Swimming
4pm	Snack, Transition from voc-hab to home	Snack, Transition from voc-hab to home	Snack, Transition from voc-hab to home	Snack, Transition from voc-hab to home	Snack, Transition from voc-hab to home	Snack, Shift transition	Snack, Shift transition
5pm	Before dinner chores	Before dinner chores	Before dinner chores	Before dinner chores	Before dinner chores	Before dinner chores	Before dinner chores

(*Continued*)

Table 3.1 Continued

TIME	MONDAY	TUESDAY	WEDNESDAY	THURSDAY	FRIDAY	SATURDAY	SUNDAY
6pm	Supper	Supper	Supper	Supper	Supper	Supper	Supper
7pm	After dinner chores	After dinner chores	After dinner chores	After dinner chores	After dinner chores	After dinner chores	After dinner chores
8pm	Evening group activity	Evening group activity	Evening group activity	Evening group activity	Evening group activity (pack lunches for hike)	Evening group activity (pack swim bags, make cookies for church)	After dinner chores
9pm	Relaxation, bed	Relaxation, bed	Relaxation, bed	Relaxation, bed	Relaxation, bed	Relaxation, bed	Relaxation, bed

*Voc-hab = vocational habilitation

resident anxious about her schedule, began her day at the barn by writing and rewriting her schedule for the day and reviewing it with a staff member, who with great patience allowed this exercise to consume the first hour of her workday. Alex, a day participant, began his day by having a staff member review his daily schedule, while Alex was doing a ritualistic hand slapping. This process was repeated over and over as Alex tried to process how the day would proceed. Another staff member spent some time helping a participant understand that her schedule included an appointment and that she would be leaving soon. Even as the participant got in the car, the staff member very sweetly explained again where she was going, what would happen, and when she would return. These examples demonstrate just a few ways in which staff assist the Bittersweet residents and day participants in understanding what they will be experiencing and doing during the day. Staff support throughout this process is a critical component of meaning and purpose at Bittersweet Farms. The success of this process requires understanding and skill on the part of staff. Also required are great patience and kindness.

There is flexibility in developing each person's schedule. Participants choose which work areas they like, often splitting the day between two areas of interest. As time passes, participants may tire of certain activities and ask to work in a different area. Beth, a long-term participant, has worked in all the different areas at Bittersweet. She enjoyed weaving and woodworking, but over time lost interest in those activities and now prefers to work in groundskeeping, mowing the lawns with a tractor mower and splitting wood. Her work has also involved maintaining machinery and fixing computers.

Self-determination is always a consideration in planning a participant's schedule. The process involves allowing participants to make choices. The multiple options for meaningful work in a wide variety of areas at Bittersweet Farms give participants many opportunities to make choices and exercise self-determination.

The schedules are person-centered, in that they are formulated to accommodate an individual's strengths as well as interests. For example, many people with ASD have strong receptive communication skills and weak expressive communication skills. A schedule designed to accommodate an individual with strong receptive skills may utilize pictures for visual support. For an individual with visual deficits or visual processing dysfunction, auditory support (recordings) might be used.

The benefits of using detailed schedules apply to both staff and residents. The schedule outlines a clear agenda and offers an opportunity for evaluating one's performance on any given task. For participants, the schedule provides additional "structured support"—a way to visually anticipate and then "cross something off a list," contributing to success and a sense of accomplishment.

Schedules can also help residents understand the purpose of an activity. For this, "if/then" scenarios are included. The if/then statement might relate to the outcome of an activity or a personal benefit for the resident. For example, for a baking activity, the statement might be worded as "If you knead the bread, we can put it in the loaf pan." A slight change in wording can focus on the outcome and add an incentive, as in "If you knead the bread, we can eat the bread after it bakes." From a program perspective, it's important to consider the projected outcome when choosing if/then statements.

Person-centeredness is also an important consideration in choosing outcome statements. Just as a young person entering adulthood chooses a career path that accommodates his or her own strengths and interests, a

Individual Schedule

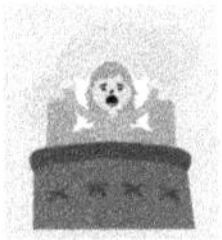	**Time to get up**
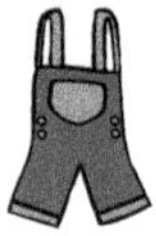	**Get dressed**
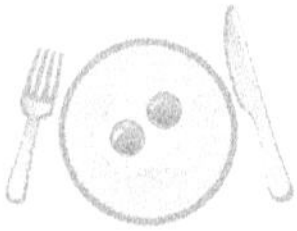	**Eat breakfast**
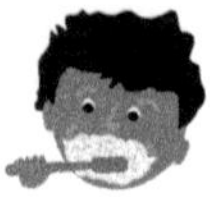	**Brush your teeth**
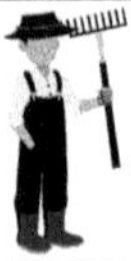	**Go to work**

Figure 3.1 Individual Schedule of Activities Depicted in Two Columns Matching Pictures to the Activity.

schedule or program for a resident at Bittersweet should incorporate that individual's strengths and interests.

Another issue to be considered in planning schedules and activities relates to differing levels of ability. While the outcome of a bread baking activity may be the same for several residents (eating the bread), the process needs to accommodate different abilities. Thus, one resident may do the measuring of the ingredients, while another resident pours the ingredients into a bowl. From woodworking, to caring for animals, to harvesting produce, the structure of the program is designed to provide opportunities for different levels of participation. Individual schedules should be detailed enough to specify the specific role an individual will play in the activity.

INDIVIDUALIZATION

Susan entered the Bittersweet program at the age of 22. The greatest concern at the time related to her aggressive and unpredictable behavior. Susan's significant behavior problems included hyperactivity, screeching, hostility, and body and hand slapping. Her language and fine motor skills were limited.

Susan had been in a sheltered workshop prior to coming to Bittersweet. Living at the farm was a positive change for her. She liked being outdoors and being physically active. Initially, a staff member accompanied her to different areas around the farm to determine which areas she could participate in. When encouraged to participate, however, she would throw herself on the ground or floor and have a temper tantrum.

To accommodate for Susan's very short attention span, staff offered hand-over-hand prompting to help her with daily work assignments. Every effort was made to keep her with consistent staff. The flexible schedule and staff understanding of her special needs allowed Susan to move from one vocational area to another until she could find an area that interested her. Eventually, working with animals and engaging in other farm activities involving gross motor skills allowed Susan to be productive.

Within two years of entering the program, Susan's behavior improved dramatically. Her self-injurious behavior and aggressive behaviors toward others greatly decreased. Her productivity improved; and with close supervision, she could persist with uncomplicated tasks, such as shucking corn. Susan also understood that the shucked corn would be put in a grinder and then used in bird feeders. Understanding the purpose of her activity increased her motivation to complete the task.

While Susan's limited fine motor skills kept her from being successful in art activities, she found enjoyment and relaxation in outdoor recreational activities, such as walking and hiking. This outdoor exercise also gives her the sensory stimulation she needs to remain calm.

Sensory Processing

The input we receive through our senses (hearing, feeling, smelling, tasting, and seeing) helps us understand and perceive the world around us. This input can draw us toward or send us reeling away from situations, depending upon the intensity of and personal association with the sensation.

Imagine sitting in a lecture hall and a bee begins flying around your head. If you don't mind bees, you might be fascinated by the miracle of flight and you might lose track of the lecture content as you observe the bee hovering over you and around the person in front of you. If you had been painfully stung in the past, you may fidget a bit and wave your arms around to discourage the bee from landing on you or anyone else nearby. You may lose track of the lecture content due to the bee floating in your personal space. If you are seriously allergic to bee stings, your response may be one closer to fear—a bit more immediate and dramatically reactive. Quickly, you may get up to leave the area, intently watching the bee's movements. You may start reaching for an anti-bee sting medication. The lecture content isn't the important issue. Safety and security are foremost. Casual observers may not understand your anxiety, not seeing the bee and not appreciating your concerns.

People with sensory disorders can be easily overwhelmed by or unresponsive to sensation. Sensory processing deficits are a well-documented hallmark of autism; yet the manner in which people with autism react to stimuli varies (Gonthier et al., 2016). Some have hyper (elevated) sensitivity with intense responses to stimuli such as light or sounds. Others have hypo (under-responsive) sensitivity to sensory input, as in a lack of awareness of extreme heat or cold.

People with autism who are hypersensitive may engage in self-stimulatory behaviors to suppress the pain or calm themselves down. People with autism who are hyposensitive may seek sensory stimulation from the outside. In working with people with ASD, it's important to understand the function their responses to sensory stimulation serves. Once this is understood, more appropriate behaviors serving the same function can be introduced. Staff working with people with autism must be aware of sensory causative factors and plan to avoid or mitigate situations where these may occur.

THE BREAD BAKER

Larry found satisfaction in baking bread. An upgrade to the Bittersweet kitchen facilities included the purchase of a commercial mixer. At the same time, Larry began to show a lack of interest in baking bread. When encouraged to continue, he would become agitated and refuse. At first, the staff thought he had simply lost interest in baking bread. Efforts to introduce other tasks in the kitchen area failed. By eliminating the possible causes of his distress, they determined he was reacting to the high-pitched whine of the new mixer. Larry was given a noise-reducing headset to wear. When he no longer heard the sound of the mixer, he was able to resume his role as the bread baker.

Structure: Designing a "Prosthetic Environment"

A prosthetic environment for people with autism has two basic elements: structure and consistency. If well designed, the environment fosters a sense of confidence and security. A prosthetic environment provides accommodations and assistive supports which facilitate understanding and reduce anxiety.

DANELLE'S SCHEDULE

Individualized visual supports clearly outlining a schedule or routine to follow throughout the day help reduce anxiety and smooth transitions from one activity to the next. Visual supports may be written or presented in pictorial format, based on the individual need for clarity regarding the routine and how the individual processes information.

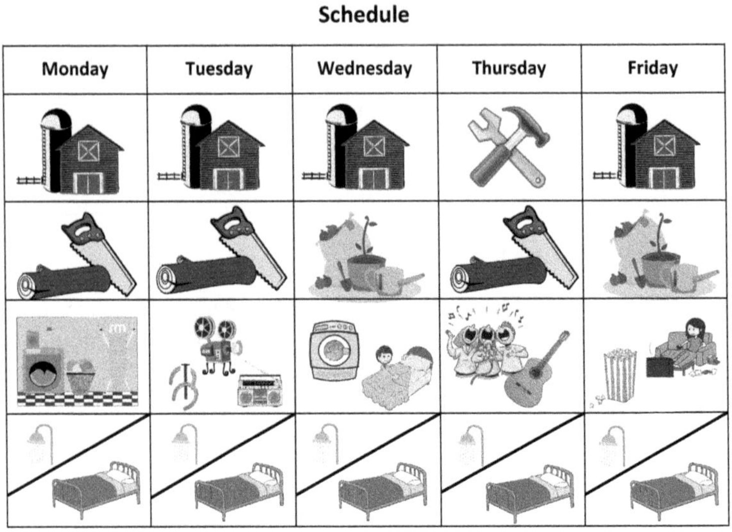

Schedule

Monday	Tuesday	Wednesday	Thursday	Friday

Figure 3.2 Danelle's Schedule.

Visitors walking around the buildings at Bittersweet may see written and pictorial instructions for even the smallest tasks such as handwashing. These detailed instructions give a sequence of simple steps to provide structure to the task and the environment.

To help us understand the importance of a supportive environment for people with ASD, David Holmes (1990) asks us to

> imagine a person without a leg who is fitted with a prosthetic limb. With a well-fitted prosthesis designed for her or his physique and activity level, this person may be able to participate in activities not physically possible otherwise. The brace may give the individual a level of independence, capability and even confidence that she or he may not be able to demonstrate without this support.

So it is for a person with autism. The prosthetic supports are routine schedules, visual cues, structured task sequences, and consistent responses from knowledgeable family, friends, and providers of services. Such "bracing"—designed to the specific qualities of the individual—provides a level of independence and success that the person may not be able to

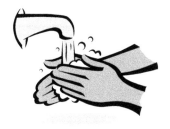

HAND WASHING PROCEDURE

1. Run hands under very warm water
2. Lather with soap
3. Scrub nails with fingernail brush (optional)
4. Rub hands together for 20 seconds, making sure to get between fingers, thumbs, wrists and forearms
5. Rinse with hot water
6. Dry hands with clean paper towel
7. Use paper towel to turn water off and open the door
8. Dispose of paper towel in the trash can

Figure 3.3 Handwashing Procedures.

achieve otherwise. Most of us would never consider asking a person who uses a prosthetic leg to attempt ambulatory tasks with no support or adaptive device. Yet, this kind of disregard often occurs with individuals with autism when their "prosthetic structure" is not followed. Either there is no structured plan suited to the individual or it may have been faded out or abandoned without direct recognition of its effectiveness.

Perhaps one of the most glaring examples of this occurs when a young person transitions from a school-age program to adult services. This can be a difficult period for any adolescent, but for those with autism the impact can be devastating, as the prosthetic supports that enable him or her to function in a school setting are no longer available.

THE TRANSITION

Josh had been enrolled in a well-designed program for students with autism. He was used to having a concise, visual schedule of pictured activities for his day. A familiar paraprofessional guided him through the steps of his class activities. Adjustments to his routine were discussed ahead of time to address anxiety over changes. Life at school was structured, well supported, and considered his sensory needs, special interests, and developing skills. Then he graduated and was assigned to the next stage of services. The supports that had been supplied in the school were no longer available or well communicated. He was in a different location, with different people, and a different schedule not suited to his sensory needs. There were limited resources and knowledge about autism to supply the individualized support he required for independence and success. His comfort level, independence, and capacity to self-control crumbled. In a way, his prosthetic supports had been yanked away from him. He would huddle in a corner, scream, and throw things at kindhearted efforts to provide direction. His achievements of the past were hidden under his responses to the stress and his loss of control.

Consistency

Solidifying participant understanding and learning requires consistency in the way information is provided and individual needs are met. Many participants in the Bittersweet program have a number of supporters across the different venues of their daily lives: their home, work, therapy, and school/vocational settings. The more individuals involved in providing services, the greater the potential for inconsistency.

Bittersweet staff depend on written information for guidance on how best to meet the needs of each individual participant. They can access this information through case files, individual service plans, and behavior support plans. While this information is important and valuable in determining the appropriate level of support, it's the details of daily events and interactions that can be the most helpful.

Ideally, communications between providers occur on a daily basis. This need not be a formal verbal or written exchange. A simple "communication book" used between service settings and providers can work wonders in providing daily information that is vital to successful outcomes.

Communications, however, can be made ineffective through certain "pitfalls." Slang, innuendo, sarcasm, and puns, in addition to not being understood, can send unintended messages. Further difficulties may

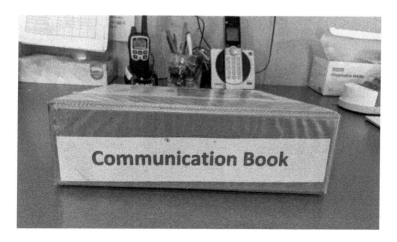

Figure 3.4 A Communication Book Is Critical in Sharing Information about Residents.

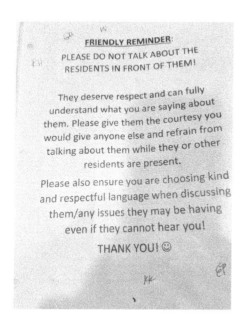

Figure 3.5 Scripts and Reminders Help the Staff Communicate to Residents in a Positive and Supportive Manner.

occur when individuals have sources of anxiety for which they seek affirmation in response. Because of this, it is often helpful to give "scripts" for all supporters to use so that the consistency and accuracy of messages are more likely assured.

The Structured Environment

Creating an appropriate environment involves more than simply designing the physical space. A structured environment incorporates defined order and sequence. It also includes expectations that are clearly, visually identified. The physical environment itself becomes a guide and support, matching the unique qualities of the individual with autism.

Constructing a prosthetic environment requires some everyday accommodations and assistive supports. A guiding principle at Bittersweet is the Ben Franklin quote, "A place for everything; everything in its place."

Work areas are prone to disorder. Use of templates, labels, and illustrations for the placement of materials, and bins, baskets, or bordered areas to contain individual work can minimize this problem. Providing a consistent location for parts or finished products can help residents

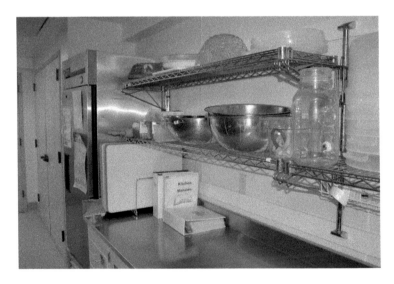

Figure 3.6 The Kitchen Is Kept Organized so that Residents Can Easily See What They Need To Use.

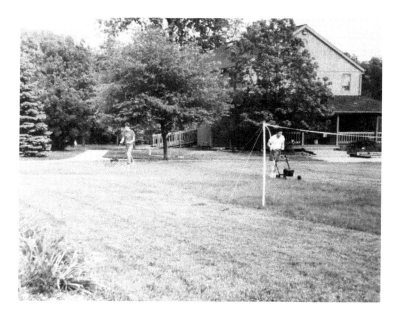

Figure 3.7 Two Residents Mow Different Segments of a Large Lawn.

maintain a better focus on their tasks. It also helps to arrange physical materials and space in a clear sequence of use.

Bittersweet has many acres of grass. The task of "mowing the yard" is far less daunting when it is divided into clearly outlined segments. To define a specific area for cutting, a staff member mows the parameter around the area as a visual boundary. Clearly outlining the boundary for a task fosters both cooperation and success. The size of the area to be mowed can be increased gradually as the person succeeds and learns the occupation. The same strategy is used for vacuuming, with small bits of paper or debris scattered to define the area to be cleaned. Establishing clear and logical boundaries removes confusion or ambiguity.

Proximity to others, sensory sensitivities, individual preferences and needs—these are factors that should be considered in designing a supportive environment. The following questions might be helpful in identifying accommodations to be made for an individual.

Does the person need a chair that moves or "floats" or a sitting ball to achieve some muscle input without having to get out of the chair to work or to attend to a task?

Would the individual do better standing or walking frequently?

Does she or he need space away from others due to concerns about being bumped or touched?

Does the person have any sensitivity to sound, lighting, or fragrances that needs to be addressed?

Many people with autism have co-existing challenges of attention deficit, organizational problems, and difficulty with behavioral self-management. With clearly defined work areas and materials, and with reduced sensory distraction, many people with ASD demonstrate more advanced skills.

SIMPLE ELIMINATE THE DISTRACTION

Janelle is compelled to rip off the flaps of cardboard boxes when there are boxes in her work area. This distraction keeps her from starting any assigned task. By keeping her work area free of cardboard boxes, she can concentrate on the job and be successful in completing her task.

Predictability

Most of us have experienced the feeling of uncertainty and confusion when given a task with no directions. Think of opening a box filled with dozens of pieces without any visual pictures as to the product to be built or instructions about how to proceed.

Understanding the sequence and the expected end product of an activity is a basic need for all of us. For people with autism, it is a critical ingredient for success. People with autism need to clearly understand the expected outcome of an activity and the step-by-step process for achieving it. Generalizing from one context to another can be very difficult for them.

Predictability is an anchor for people with autism. If an activity changes, even slightly, the sequence must be reviewed and supported (Giddan & Obee, 1996). One of the challenges for Bittersweet staff is establishing day-to-day and week-to-week familiarity for the residents who are easily unsettled by unexpected change.

One of the advantages of the Bittersweet Farms setting is the way in which it allows residents to naturally observe changes in seasons as they occur. These changes occur gradually, while many elements of the environment remain consistent. Staff continually work to create an awareness of the physical changes each season brings. This effort enhances the residents' understanding of time and change.

A part of structuring predictability for any given activity involves a clearly understood first step and last step. When a task is completed to a particular standard that can be seen and/or measured, the individual

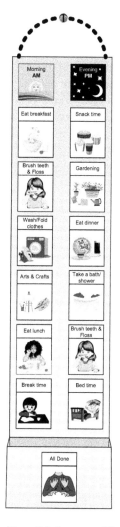

Figure 3.8 Sequence Chart.

should be able to indicate "FINISHED" in an obvious and concrete way. He or she should also have an understanding of what comes next in the sequence of the schedule. If sequences are to be repeated until all materials are exhausted, the person may do best with a "REPEAT" sign or a flip chart that shows the task starting over again.

Making quality judgments is difficult for people with autism. While they may be able to follow a sequence, they may not be able to consider changes that alter the outcome.

UNDERSTANDING OUTCOMES

During a routine check of Jim's living quarters, staff found all of Jim's clothes neatly folded and put away in their appropriate drawers. However, the clothing was wet. Jim followed the sequence for washing, drying, and folding his laundry. What he did not consider was that the dryer had malfunctioned and had no heat. So even though he was successful in the task, the results were not.

Structured Flexibility

Despite our best intentions, life does not always unfold as planned. Perhaps the road you are taking to get to the store is closed for repair, or once you get to the store you find out that the item you want is sold out. Preparing participants for change is a strategic part of proactive planning. The concept of "structured flexibility" plays a role in this process. Structured flexibility provides a framework for "going with the flow" while still maintaining structure.

Because of their need for predictability, helping residents learn to cope with changing variables is a constant challenge. The goal is to secure confidence in the outcomes and focus on the positives. This can be prepared for in advance by creating situations that require flexibility and by demonstrating flexibility in the face of a dilemma. The process involves respectful and empathic communication to describe what is occurring, to highlight the positives within the situation, and to assure desired outcomes.

Structure gives an individual assurance of what is going to occur, not just at that moment, but also throughout the course of the day. If one element in the sequence breaks down, this may lead to confusion and

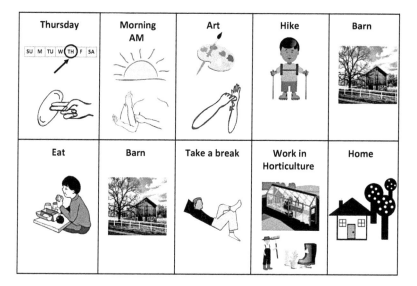

Figure 3.9 Visual Schedule with Picture Cards.

anxiety about the rest of the day's events. Consider, for example, a scenario where a resident understands that, after he goes to the barber shop, he can go to a store to purchase needed items and then return home and complete his usual daily routine which ends with watching his favorite TV show. If the barber shop is closed, the resident may become doubtful that any of the other daily events will occur. He may thus become agitated and confused. He needs the assurance that even though he won't get his hair cut, the rest of the day's events can still occur. A visual schedule with picture cards can be useful in this situation, as pictured events can be rearranged when unplanned disruptions occur. The resident can see that, in spite of one change, the structure and routine of the rest of the day persist.

At times, something in the environment presents the need for flexibility. At other times, it might be something within the individual. Perhaps the individual becomes ill, has to use the bathroom, or doesn't want to do what is on the schedule. The ability to be flexible in such situations expresses empathic concern and can avoid power struggles.

The key to success is to find a careful balance between structure and flexibility, so that one is not sacrificed for the other. Not every situation lends itself well to flexibility. Yet, there may be times when a situation is so chaotic that maintaining structure becomes extremely difficult. The aim is to provide structure as needed, to the best extent possible. The tools of persuasion, negotiation, and compromise can be used to help maintain an appropriate balance between structure and flexibility.

The strategies employed require careful planning. After something occurs causing even a slight change in routine, a plan should be in place to allow for a smooth transition back to the original format. The following guidelines can be helpful in such situations.

1.   Choose a situation or activity that is pleasurable and in which the person feels comfortable and relaxed.
2.   Introduce the change as gradually as the individual can manage and be aware of the effect that the change may have on the person.
3.   Offer structured choices within the environment or situation that enable the individual to choose an option as independently as possible.

Communication: A Multifaceted Approach

In addition to structuring the physical environment, interactions between residents and staff can also be structured. Often, a person with communication challenges may revert to inappropriate physical assertions or unsuccessful repetitive verbal expressions in an effort to get his or her needs met. By building a rich communicative environment and routine that taps into the person's skills, and by teaching and supporting successful communication alternatives with consistency, the staff can promote more effective communication.

COMMUNICATION: A MULTIFACETED APPROACH

Daryl is non-verbal and needs communication support through the use of sign language and through pictured schedules and task sequences. However, he has difficulty manipulating his fingers for some sign language movements. Staff are aware of how Daryl adjusts sign language to express his basic needs. They recognize his body language indicating anxiety, and they are familiar with his preferences and daily habit patterns. They provide him with a regular routine to follow in which he can take some control and in which he practices successful communication methods. Staff offer him alternate ways to make requests or decisions by routinely having him select objects, point to pictured choices, and by modeling sign language to represent his interests. Daryl is encouraged to carry pictured messages between work areas so that he can request materials as he needs them. Using the pictured messages allows Daryl to experience the power of using effective communication options. Daryl uses a computer to make his own pictured lists of things to gather for a job or for items needed on a grocery list. He also chooses from a pictured communication list to indicate his needs and interests to others. Daryl's schedule has pictured activity options on separate cards so he can select what he would like to do and in the order he prefers.

Structuring social interaction at the individual's preferred mode and level of ability is an important part of the daily routine. Shared experiences during such interactions allow relationships to grow fluidly and meaningfully. Structuring social interactions can involve establishing a format for successful greetings and providing scripts for specific communicative exchanges. Scripts can provide appropriate methods for refusing, requesting, responding, and reacting. Structuring social interactions can help residents comprehend familiar instructions and encourage them to become more independent and successful in expressing their needs and wants.

REACHING OUT

Karen used to grab the hands of people near her, unpredictably and firmly. She did not distinguish between a friend and a stranger. She seemed to like the feel of the hands. At Bittersweet, she was encouraged to greet staff by extending her hand for a handshake. With consistent cues from those she met, she learned to verbally request "Handshake please" rather than just grabbing someone's hand. She also learned to accept the fact that sometimes people did not want a handshake!

EXAMPLE OF SCRIPTED COMMUNICATION CUES

I want a drink please.	I have a headache.
I want to eat please.	I am hungry.
I want music please.	I am angry.
I want bathroom please.	I am hot.
I want a break please.	I am cold.
I want a head rub please.	I am sick.
I want a cold cloth please.	
I want a pillow please.	
I want to rest please.	
I want outside please.	
I want inside please.	
I want medicine please.	
I want an arm squeeze please.	

The word "autism" stems from the Greek words *autos* ("self") and *ismos* ("state"). The term was coined in 1912 by Swiss psychiatrist Paul Bleuler (1857–1939), to describe a condition of abnormal self-absorption characterized by lack of response to other humans and by limited ability or disinclination to communicate (Resnick, 2017). This description continues to characterize the classic diagnosis for autism today. Difficulties in social interactions and communication and tendencies to self-isolate and focus on repetitive and restrictive patterns of thought and behaviors are all part of the syndrome known as autism. Bittersweet addresses these characteristics by providing opportunities for residents to experience real-life experiences in simulated situations, practicing scripted responses that enable appropriate social interactions. As residents' skills develop, they are able to successfully interact in the greater community.

Residents at Bittersweet have an opportunity to shop at the Bittersweet store. There, they can purchase things they need (such as deodorants and toothpaste) or want (such as books and chewing gum) using their own money. The store is stocked with items listed on residents' "want lists." The "STORE OPEN" dates are circled on individual calendars and are eagerly anticipated by the residents. In addition to the social interactions this activity provides, purchasing items at the store also promotes an understanding of how money and budgeting work.

Visual Supports

In a residential setting or facility where there are differing staff shifts and a variety of group activities, it is imperative that all staff follow the same sequence of events and established patterns of interactions. Visual supports are essential aids for staff. Minor differences between how staff model, verbalize, or present a task can cause great confusion and frustration for persons with cognitive and/or social challenges. Clear visual instructions can minimize these problems.

Visual supports are often essential aids for residents, as well. While visual cues help most of us process information, they are imperative for people with autism. Dr Temple Grandin, perhaps one of the most well-known individuals on the spectrum, describes her thought process as "thinking in pictures" and even describes a visual file folder for storing categories of information (Grandin, 2006).

Visual support can take many forms: room arrangement, tangible objects, reproduction samples, color photos, black-and-white images, life-like drawings, colored line drawings, black-and-white line drawings, words, symbols. Helping a person with autism to understand the representative or associated meaning of the visual support is key to success. These supports can be very simple, functional communication tools or very complex, interpretive devices.

The nature of the item or image needed as a visual support is dictated by the cognitive level and interest of the individual for whom the system is developed and the resources and creativity of the crafter.

Fading Supports

People with autism do not graduate or "age-out" as they grow into adulthood. The need for some supports may actually intensify as the transition from the routine structure of school merges into the uncertain regrouping of adult services. Different people, different places, and completely different routines will develop a different pattern of responses. Unexpected occurrences that may be invigorating surprises to some people may be highly challenging or even distressing to persons with autism. A new, unfamiliar activity, although seemingly fun, may not be positive. Many people with ASD have difficulty translating understandings and skills from one situation to another. While they may be successful in completing routines in a familiar setting, they may not be able to do so in other settings and situations.

While it's important to develop and encourage a person's independence and capabilities, some individuals with autism need lifelong support in certain areas. An analogy to consider is a corrective lens for visual problems. The specific measurements and form of the corrective lens may change through the years based on the person's growth, development, and interests. The prescription is changed to meet the special needs of the individual. Without this visual support even pleasurable activities like reading a story, watching a favorite television show, or going to a movie may elevate stress levels to the point of discomfort and irritability. Some persons with autism will need specific supports throughout their lifetime; others may need a specific support for only a period of time. Hopefully, those required "guides" will evolve with the growth and changes of the individual, just like eyewear.

Sufficient balance is an important aspect of support. Understanding when and how much support can be withdrawn after an individual has made successful transitions is a major consideration. This is a decision that should be made with the individual and with those who know the person well in accordance with objective observation and assessment.

People with autism tend to have a special appreciation and need for routine and consistency. A supported structure and confidence in a regular schedule are often a salve that soothes rough edges. With the right, individualized structure, the route may be travelled with greater success and quality of life experienced. Laying the foundation of structure and support is a critical first step on the journey. Once this is in place, the next steps can be taken.

References

Giddan, J. J., & Obee, V. L. (1996). Adults with autism: Rehabilitation challenges and practices. *Journal of Rehabilitation, 6*(2), 72–76.

Gonthier, C., Longuépée, L., & Bouvard, M. (2016). Sensory processing in low-functioning adults with autism spectrum disorder: Distinct sensory profiles and their relationships with behavioral dysfunction. *Journal of Autism and Developmental Disorders, 46*(9), 3078–3089.

Grandin, T., & Sacks, O. (2006). *Thinking in pictures, expanded edition: My life with autism.* New York: Vintage Press.

Holmes, D. L. (1990). Community-based services for children and adults with autism: The Eden family of programs. *Journal of Autism and Developmental Disorders, 20*(3), 339–351.

Resnick, J. (2017). Paul Eugen Bleuler (1857–1939). *Embryo Project Encyclopedia* (2017-04-06). ISSN: 1940-5030. http://embryo.asu.edu/handle/10776/11464

4   The Road to Community

Partnership and Purpose

Bittersweet is built on a cooperative relationship between staff and residents that requires mutual support and collaborative side-by-side job sharing. This approach is in contrast with the traditional "teacher–student model." Partnership, a core value of the program, builds on the need to increase the social and emotional reciprocity of the residents. In all activities, staff at Bittersweet strive to be supportive and facilitating—not managerial.

Every activity at Bittersweet has a positive purpose with outcomes that can be observed and appreciated. Understanding how each person's efforts fit into the steps needed to complete a given project provides the motivation to be involved. Knowing the reason for and intended outcome of a task creates an environment for meaningful interactions and, ultimately, positive self-esteem. This chapter focuses on partnership and purpose, cornerstones of the Bittersweet approach.

Partnership

Partnership is the core of Bittersweet's program. It is the basic principle that guides all interactions and activities at Bittersweet. It is what makes Bittersweet unique. The "give and take" of social interactions fostered by sharing activities, interests, and emotional responses is an integral component of Bittersweet's intervention program. Because people with autism usually lack good eye contact, have difficulty developing peer relationships, and lack social and emotional reciprocity, the partnership component of the program provides the basis for a therapeutic process incorporated throughout the day at Bittersweet. Without partnerships, residents would remain isolated, missing the enjoyment of human interaction and unable to function as a member of the community. Belonging to a community is a critical component of quality of life.

Staff, who take responsibility for the operation, implementation, and evaluation of the Bittersweet program, are at the core of what makes

DOI: 10.4324/9781003271048-5

the program successful. What makes the Bittersweet program exceptional, however, is the equal partnership between staff and participants. Becoming an effective partner is an art requiring understanding, creativity, and an open mind.

RECIPROCAL PARTNERING

Bittersweet Farms houses horses in a barn a short distance from the main residential building. One winter afternoon, the pump at the horse barn "froze up" and water for the horses had to be carried in buckets from the main house. A staff member demonstrated the meaning of reciprocal partnership while fulfilling the duty of watering the horses. Rather than both she and the resident each individually carry a heavy bucket of water, the staff member slid a strong broomstick through the handles of the buckets. She demonstrated to a highly challenged resident how to help carry the buckets by taking one end of the broom while she took the other end.

Without a lot of verbal instruction, the two of them walked up and over the snow-covered hill to the barn. They had to carefully balance and adjust the load to keep the buckets from spilling! It was a remarkable choreography of silent coordination. Upon successfully arriving at the barn, both partners demonstrated a sense of accomplishment and teamwork with smiles and high fives! The mundane act of watering the horses provided a teachable moment of successful partnership, interdependence, and cooperation.

Morton Ann Gernsbacher, a specialist in autism and psycholinguistics, has devoted a great deal of her research efforts to the cognitive and neurological processes of people with autism. She encourages reciprocity when working with people with autism spectrum disorder (ASD) and describes it as a mutual, symmetrical exchange that occurs when neither party is in a dominant position (Gernsbacher, 2006). The partnership model implemented at Bittersweet reflects this understanding of reciprocity. However, for the process to be effective in increasing social interactions, it needs to be purposeful, planned, and developed by staff. The professionals initiate the interaction, pay attention to what interests a resident, share that interest, and then follow the lead of the resident to establish a reciprocal relationship. This type of partnership does not just occur. It must be taught.

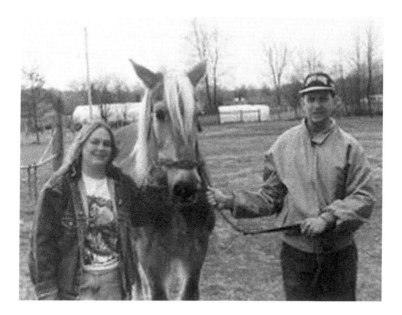

Figure 4.1 Tammy Bolley-Chambers in Partnership with a Resident Walking a Horse.

Another important aspect of the partnership approach relates to how staff and others view the residents and activities at Bittersweet. Residents are not viewed as patients or students. They're viewed as partners or co-workers. The services provided at Bittersweet aren't attempts to "fix" the residents. The focus is on enhancing quality of life. Staff and residents work together on constructive activities that offer satisfaction and joy in completing something of value.

Partnership and Communication

The speech and language therapist evaluates each resident's needs at the time of admission to Bittersweet. The therapist first does intensive individual work with the resident and then develops a plan which is taught to the staff. The staff then use the recommended language and communication techniques during partnership activities. This approach is so much more efficient than a resident seeing the speech therapist for an appointment each week!

Vocabulary, language concepts, and communication skills are taught throughout each day during every partnership activity. Consultation with the speech therapist is ongoing so that skills continue to progress and can be tailored to intervention as needed. Encouraging residents to talk about feelings and ask for what is needed reduces frustration and aggression. This approach can only happen in a partnership relationship where reciprocal interaction is the goal. Expressive and receptive communication levels are updated each year and placed in a binder for the staff to use as a guide. The following is an example of an entry made in 2021 about Chuck's expressive language skills:

> Chuck is verbal and can often express his wants and needs. He will initiate conversation, but the content is concrete, self-oriented, and anchored in familiar people. Chuck answers questions using phrases or simple sentences. At times he may say 'no' when the answer he really intends to say is 'yes.' This may relate to another unresolved concern or topic which needs to be addressed first before that question. He is unable to apply language to social situations appropriately; he does not maintain eye contact and does not observe the cues of moods or feelings of others.

The following entry describes Chuck's expressive language skills:

> Chuck is receptive to verbal one- and two-step directions, although he has a short attention span and a slight delay in language processing. Using a visual picture schedule at the beginning of each shift may help Chuck's understanding of the day's events and aid in his participation.

A review of the residents' records indicated that only 4 of the 20 residents included in the program evaluation were rated as having no problems with limited expressive language when they were admitted to Bittersweet. Eleven were rated as having severe problems. Seven of the residents showed improvement by one or more levels by 2021, when the study was completed. Deficits in verbal and non-verbal communication are a central characteristic of people on the autism spectrum. Improvements in these areas are essential to reduce frustration which can lead to aggression and self-injury. Increased communication is also important for the development of interpersonal relationships.

DEVELOPING COMMUNICATION SKILLS

With direction from the speech therapist, the staff were able to help Chuck improve his communication skills within supportive real-life situations. During partnership activities, vocabulary was emphasized to help Chuck name all parts and aspects of the materials he handled. Similarities and differences between items and categorizations of objects and materials were stressed in all situations. Social language was modeled and taught. The strong partnership component of the program allowed for speech therapy to be integrated into all aspects of Chuck's vocational and social activities. Over time, this instruction has helped Chuck interact well with others and communicate his needs.

WITH HELP FROM THE SPEECH/ LANGUAGE THERAPIST

Although Victor did not initiate interaction when he was a participant, he benefited from the partnership aspect of Bittersweet. A speech and language therapist worked intently with Victor and helped the staff enhance Victor's receptive and expressive communication. Victor was deaf but had been taught some sign language over the years. He was also encouraged to use a "reality board" for storytelling that defined the weather, temperature, lunch menu, notable activities of the day, and how he was feeling. Storytelling uses sign language and simple pictures. Victor was encouraged to expand the storylines and sign in complete simple sentences or phrases. Staff were instructed to use sign language to describe activities and what was happening around the farm to help Victor understand his surroundings and anticipate what would be happening next. This speaks to the importance of a full-time speech therapist on staff!

Partnership and Leisure

Partnership extends beyond work activities to leisure activities, including art projects, music, and other recreational activities, such as card and board games. Research has shown that art therapy helps lower anxiety, facilitates attachment to caregivers, and improves social engagement in general (Durrani, 2014).

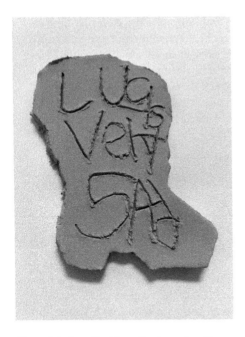

Figure 4.2 One Resident Used an Art Therapy Project to Express Her Feelings. "Lucy (Charlie Brown's Lucy) Is Very Sad." Picture by Kim Dennler.

The residents at Bittersweet enjoy music activities. Many have participated in the bell choir (pictured in Chapter 5) as well as taking private lessons on piano, guitar, drums, etc. Residents enjoy sing-alongs and will individually sing their favorite songs, such as "Our House," "I've Been Working on the Railroad," "Garden Song," and "Country Road." A study on music therapy and autism found that 40 subjects exhibited improvements in language and communication, as well as in behavioral, cognitive, musical, and perceptual motor skills after two years of music therapy (Kaplan & Steele, 2005). Working in partnership in leisure activities helps residents form attachments with staff and increases their interpersonal skills.

Partnership and Community

People with ASD have many barriers to being part of a community, such as aggression and communication deficits. Yet, being part of a community is critical for quality of life. Residents at Bittersweet develop relationships with staff who become like family. Even when staff leave the farm, many come back and visit residents or invite them to their homes for holidays and important events, such as weddings, birthday parties, and holidays. One resident was able to fly to Arizona to visit a former staff member with whom he had a close relationship. Many of the residents are involved in church communities. Staff also organize Bittersweet community activities at the farm, and everybody is included. Everyone is part of the family!

Bittersweet recently built a large fire pit with a sheltered area with seating and a large grill next to it. This is a perfect area for community gatherings and parties.

VALENTINE PARTY

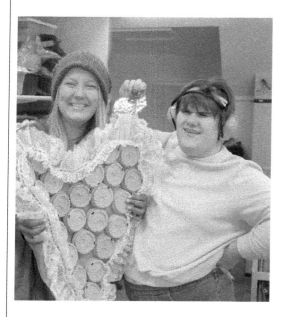

Figure 4.3 The Staff and Residents Enjoyed Planning for the Annual Valentine's Day Party. Everyone Got Dressed Up and Enjoyed the Food, Music, and Standing in Front of the Photo Board for Pictures.

KAREN

Karen became a valued part of the Bittersweet and local community. Interventions designed to help her become aware of others and to interact with peers allowed her to interact with others. Karen was often invited to have dinner with staff members and their families. She attended a baby shower and made a baby quilt as a gift. One staff member invited her to his sister's birthday party. Because of the high turnover of staff at Bittersweet, many of whom lived locally, Karen would be greeted by former staff as well as local venders when she went to town. When Karen was in hospital before she died, over 100 people came to visit her. Former staff stayed in touch to share information on her condition. Karen had made substantial gains in the domains of interpersonal relationship and social inclusion.

NATHAN

Nathan made gains in the areas of interpersonal relations and social inclusion. He had a sense of humor and bonded with some of the staff members who would engage in non-verbal games with him. He exhibited a concern for his housemates, and would complete chores and enjoy leisure trips with a small group. Rarely did he have an outburst while on outings in the community. Nathan attended a small church in the area; and after he died, the community organized a memorial service and planted a tree at Bittersweet in his honor. Clearly, Nathan was considered a part of the church community.

Apprenticeship Model

The reciprocal partnership approach used at Bittersweet is referred to as an apprenticeship model (Karst & Van Bourgondien, 1991). With this model, residents learn through demonstrations, modeling, and imitation or experience. They work side by side with staff, completing meaningful work. Because Bittersweet is grounded in an understanding of autism, flexibility is built into the structure, allowing time for residents to learn communication and social skills and to build meaningful relationships while working.

The speech and language therapist evaluates residents' needs and teaches staff language and communication techniques to use during partnership activities.

The staff help participants contribute at their individual level of ability, yet sharing tasks equally. Jobs are sequenced in such a way that persons of varying abilities can share in the steps of the activity. The functional application of a skill done in context with a trusted and supportive partner/co-worker is retained more easily than simple skill-building exercises. The apprenticeship nature of the work structure allows staff to offer a variety of tasks in a work setting where participants can become involved at their own interest and ability level. The apprenticeship model allows participants to learn new skills while observing and working along with staff.

One staff person can partner with several participants at the same time, but planning is the key. Everyone involved in the activity must know the purpose of the task at his or her level of comprehension. Each must have a specified motivation for participating. The role of staff is to ensure that each participant receives the support needed to be actively involved in the shared occupation.

WORKING IN THE WOODSHOP

The woodshop at Bittersweet is managed by skilled craftsmen who build furniture and small wooden objects. The woodshop is filled with activities at all levels, such as sanding and hammering nails, as well as working with saws and using different types of power equipment. At times, a 50-pound bag of eared corn might fulfill a participant's sensory needs by using his or her fingers to remove the corn from the cobs, putting the corn in a meat grinder, and then cranking the grinder. The cracked corn is then put in a newly built bird feeder or added to the animal grain in the barn. Another activity involves gathering wood from the wooded area on the farm, putting it in carts, and hauling it to the woodshop. For each activity, a skilled craftsperson works alongside participants at all levels, gradually teaching skills with patience and encouragement.

Engaging in creative sharing and breaking tasks into small steps require time. If the goal is simply to complete the task as quickly and efficiently as possible, this is not the approach to use. The intent at Bittersweet is to develop reciprocal interaction and interdependence.

All activities at Bittersweet are carefully planned. The partnership approach involved in digging a hole would typically start with a discussion and visual demonstration of how to use a shovel. It would include some discussion and demonstration about the size and shape of the hole that's needed. The object to be planted or erected would be inspected. The total job would be shared, reflecting a team effort, versus a "manager and worker" mentality.

USING A TWO-MAN SAW

Purpose and partnership have an important role in engaging and maintaining participants in physical activity. A prime example of this can be seen in the use of a "two-man saw." Modern tools such as a chainsaw are certainly a more efficient way to cut wood than using a chainsaw. However, there are safety concerns to be considered. The noise can also be unsettling. Additionally, using a chainsaw is a solitary activity and does not encourage engagement and reciprocity. The use of a two-man saw, on the other hand, is by design and necessity a reciprocal activity which maximizes partnership to accomplish the goal of cutting through the wood while also supplying a good amount of physical activity.

Purpose

Purpose is one of the defining characteristics of the Bittersweet model. Activities for the residents are designed to be functional and situated in a meaningful context. Activities are also designed in relation to the level of one's understanding. This model invites full involvement. Taking a walk may be a very beneficial activity for sensory needs. Building a functional reason for going on the walk—such as delivering a message, carrying trash to a dumpster, taking materials to another work site or area of the farm—provides a purpose for the walk. Providing a functional reason for an activity in a seamless way will likely lead to better and more successful outcomes.

Demonstrating and teaching, not just how something is to be accomplished but also "why" something should be done, infuse an activity with meaning or purpose. The word "meaning," in this context, is used in a proactive way. Understanding one's role in any given task is motivating and provides an impetus for cooperation on a given endeavor.

The farm is organized in ways that provide purposeful activities for residents to motivate them to do the physical work. For example, at one time, a separate garden was dedicated to growing ingredients for salsa. When the produce was harvested, the residents made salsa and enjoyed eating it. This made all the gardening worth the effort! The grapevines that are tended provide tasty snacks, produce to take to the farmers' market, and vines to make dried wreaths to sell at festivals. The horses that are cared for pull a wagon for friends and families at gatherings. The rhythm of the farm provides aerobic activities to reduce anxiety and mood disorders and provide sensory stimulation. Adding purpose and satisfaction increases the quality of life for the residents.

FROM DESTRUCTIVE TO PURPOSEFUL ACTIVITY

When Karen first moved to Bittersweet, she displayed minimal productivity and skill development. She had a limited attention span and difficulty following directions and staying on task. She also had severe outward behaviors which became violent and aggressive. Her aggressive behavior included biting, kicking, scratching, and hitting. Physical intervention was usually necessary to support her and others near her. At one time, her severe behaviors were averaging eight per month.

When Karen became agitated, staff intervened by firmly directing her to stop and asking her to return to task. Staff also asked her to indicate what was wrong. If her behavior escalated, she was offered a walk or a change of location and supervised from a distance. Karen was rewarded for being calm by being given a cup of herbal tea.

Within a few years, Karen's severe behavioral incidents decreased to the point where her behavior management program was no longer needed. While she still had an occasional outburst, she was not as aggressive. The change was attributed to the staff's ability to understand what Karen wanted or was trying to communicate through her behavior. If Karen was breaking branches off trees, staff would suggest that she pick up sticks from the ground and break them rather than breaking branches from a living tree.

Finding purposeful activities to replace Karen's compulsive behaviors took creativity on the part of staff. Over time, however, in partnership with staff, Karen was able to become more productive. She made beautiful grapevine wreaths, tea-house desserts, and art for calendars and cards. Her creative activities helped her to develop relationships and gave her a sense of pride.

By focusing on partnership and purpose, the Bittersweet model allows each individual to be recognized for his or her abilities and to experience the satisfaction of making meaning contributions to the community in which he or she lives and works. Such experiences allow the residents to enjoy a rich quality of life.

Understanding Individual Needs

A shared partnership requires each staff member to know the needs and interests of every participant. Such an understanding is a prerequisite for building a personal relationship and a working partnership. Staff need to "enter into the world" of those they serve by understanding their interests, sensory needs, and desires. Bittersweet staff are trained to develop an understanding of the values and capabilities of all the residents. Staff then build on the residents' attributes to support their learning and growth.

Each participant who enters a Bittersweet program has a well-documented medical, educational, and behavioral history. Interviews with parents and caregivers allow staff to learn participants' history of interests, gifts, sensitivities, behavioral concerns, and limits on activities involving social interaction and communication. This information, along with the results of a functional analysis of daily living skills and other initial assessments, is used to develop a behavioral development plan listing behaviors to increase and behaviors to decrease. Methods or strategies for how to do this are also detailed in the individual plan.

BEHAVIORAL MANAGEMENT PLAN

During an initial assessment and records review, the staff learned that John, a new participant, had repetitive behaviors of throwing objects and counting. As a result of staff creativity, John was asked to throw gourds into a wheelbarrow and take them to the compost to throw them in bins. John was able to count as he threw objects. Taking a partnership approach, the staff joined him with the throwing and counting and used the opportunity to take turns, encourage communication, and develop a relationship with John. John was also encouraged to throw leaves in Halloween garbage bags and place them around the farm for decoration. Despite John's restricted interests and behaviors, through a partnership intervention, he became an important team member in helping maintain the farm.

Figure 4.4 shows an individual chart developed for one resident and provides an example of how staff plan in detail how to promote a

Asa

Name of Goal: Participation   **Frequency:** 1x daily or as needed

Annual Goal: Asa will actively participate in half or more of the routine, preferred, and scheduled activities for him each shift with one verbal prompt or less for 75% of trials

Rationale: Asa requires continual assistance from staff in order to participate in daily activities and remain on task as he has a history of being withdrawn.

Projected Completion: 7/20

Staff will offer Asa choices of preferred and routine activities to develop an individualized schedule together at the beginning of each waking shift. Asa typically prefers to write down his schedule with paper and pencils.	When offering choices, staff will be sure to offer Asa at least 2 preferred recreational activities (see attached activity plan), allowing Asa to choose at least one to participate in for the shift.	Staff will review the schedule with him throughout the day to assure him what to aspect and for what to prepare.	Staff will encourage Asa to be physically active and participate in preferred activities, as well as house duties.

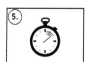

Staff will give Asa timelines throughout the shift and prompt and check up on him periodically to ensure follow through.	Staff will provide Asa positive attention and engage him in conversations meaningful to him.	Staff will explain the purpose and value of activities to Asa in ways he can understand with hopes to motivate his participation.	Don't forget to document accordingly on CareTracker!

Figure 4.4 Asa's Schedule.

desired skill or behavior. The goal, in this case, is to help the resident actively participate in scheduled activities. As illustrated, the plan includes opportunities for Asa to make choices, to be physically active, to understand the purpose of an activity, and to enjoy the experience of success.

Understanding the Process

Respect, appreciation, and tolerance for process seem to be an increasingly rare phenomenon. This may be due, in large part, to advances in technology and a culture obsessed with efficiency and multitasking. But for the partnership approach to work, an appreciation of the process must be intertwined in all aspects of teaching and doing. Being aware of and realistic about the time required for long-term success cannot be overemphasized. There are many variables on the journey. Sometimes, in our enthusiasm, we aim for big strides. Examples of this can be seen in matching people with community employment and/or social groups and activities before the necessary skill development has taken place.

THE RESTAURANT SCENE

Phillip wanted to work as a waiter in a restaurant. Although he possessed the skills required, (e.g., writing orders, delivering food without spilling, and entering information into a cash register), Phil had difficulty with the necessary social skills. On a typical day, certain aspects of customer service, such as greeting and making small talk, were challenges. On a "bad" day, Phil might say and do things that could be received as rude or offensive. Given the importance of customer service for the restaurant owners, it is highly likely that even 1 bad day out of 365 could jeopardize employment. It could also be hurtful for Phil by adding a sense of failure and rejection, projecting a shadow on future endeavors. Phil worked toward his goal by serving as a waiter at Bittersweet, simulating a restaurant experience. Currently, he is employed at a local restaurant several days a week. Although he still has social issues incompatible with his stated goal of being a waiter, he finds satisfaction in other restaurant roles to which he is assigned.

BOWLING

Bowling is an activity at Bittersweet that many enjoy. One resident, an avid bowler, asked if she could participate in a "regular" league. This individual was very capable, conscientious, and had excellent verbal skills. She worked well independently with tasks requiring little social interaction. Staff assisted in locating a league for her to join. Although her bowling proficiency was never questioned, her social behaviors proved to be a serious impediment. Even with ongoing staff support, her incessant chatting and inappropriate comments created friction with teammates. Continuing participation in the league was not feasible. However, the experience provided her with insights that have proven to be valuable in daily interactions with others at Bittersweet. She continues to bowl with other residents and takes pride in her ability.

Bittersweet staff focus on providing direction and feedback in a way that is constructive, supportive, and immediate. They work from the premise that "bad" days should never be overlooked and that they should always have a backup plan.

Activity Planning

The greater the number of persons requiring support from a single staff member, the more difficult it is to develop partnership objectives and meaningful engagement. Sometimes, the ratios are dictated by circumstance but more often by funding. Regardless of the driving cause, the greater the number of people needing support, the more critical planning and proactive strategies become. Keeping a group of individuals actively engaged and providing the appropriate structural supports are challenges that need to be addressed during activity planning and implementation. The situation requires staff to know the individual characteristics of each person in the group and have a solid understanding of how to interact effectively with each one.

Two principles underscore all planning: (1) adhere to daily routines with as few deviations as possible as a baseline for planning activities; and (2) have supports, including materials and information about the participants, available in advance. The partnership system will only work if time is devoted to detailed preparation.

Sometimes a "great idea" for an activity is pursued with all good intention without the array of important details being considered. It may seem like a nice idea to take someone who loves music to the Rock & Roll Hall of Fame Museum. However, before this decision is made, there are basic factors to consider. First, consider the individual. Examine what is known about this person and walk through the course of the day to predict how it will go. Does the individual tolerate long car rides? Who else is going and do they enjoy each other's company? What are the potential sensory stimulations at the museum and how will the individual process them? What accommodations can be made? How will the individual handle a change to his or her daily schedule and structure? How long will the individual be able to enjoy the museum? What food will be available, and will it be liked? Others who have interacted with and supported the individual should be consulted. The knowledge and experience they can share may be invaluable.

VICTOR

Victor could be easily overstimulated. An example of why this needs to be understood occurred after Detroit Redwings tickets were donated to Bittersweet and Victor and several other residents attended. After 15 minutes, Victor was in such a state of sensory overload that the group had to leave. Victor would have been better off out in nature with activities which provided the kind of sensory stimulation he needed!

Staff Considerations

At the center of every successful endeavor are staff responsible for the operation, implementation, and evaluation of its program. Therefore, attention must be given to the recruitment, selection, training, monitoring, and evaluation of employees.

Role of Staff

All Bittersweet employees, including administrative staff, are expected to be co-workers in the daily activities at the farm. Employees never question whether or not to participate in a specific task—be it a jog through the farm or cleaning the stables—as participation is a given. Staff realize that through the participation process comes understanding and learning.

Staff also know that looking for the ABILITY versus the DIS-ability of each person is required in order to build on the individual's gifts and/or interests. They thus make it a priority to get to know each participant well so that they use this information to build meaningful relationships.

Individual job descriptions include not only primary work assignments, such as horticulture or housekeeping, but also details outlining roles and responsibilities relating to the implementation of the Bittersweet philosophy and model.

BITTERSWEET INC. POSITION DESCRIPTION

Position Title: Direct support professional (DSP)
Date: 12/2015
Reports to: Program leader and manager
Position Purpose:

The direct support professional must implement Bittersweet's philosophy and approach focusing on meaning and motivation, aerobic activity, partnership and purpose, and structure and support. He or she must work to foster positive relationships with residents and staff by continually upholding dignity, respect, and kindness. Priding oneself on recognizing the unique qualities and needs of each individual with autism and addressing those needs appropriately are a necessary aspect in acting out the position of direct support professional.

The direct support professional is responsible to work at maximizing quality of life by providing teaching, choices, and activities, and by giving personal attention and engagement to the participants of Bittersweet. He or she must work to ensure the health and safety of participants while providing an environment that fosters both growth and development. This position will also be asked to respectfully perform all additional duties as assigned by supervisors.

Qualifications:

- Minimum of a high school education or GED.
- Prefer one to two years' experience working with individuals with autism and/or other developmental disabilities.

- Valid driver's license along with eligibility to be insured.

Essential functions of position: All of the essential job functions listed below are necessary in order to effectively perform the job.

- Behavior should be professional at all times and consistent with Bittersweet's culture, mission, core values, philosophy, and policies and procedures, including treating participants with dignity and respect.
- Promote communication, choice, independence, socialization, and empowerment for the participants.
- Work in partnership with participants in assigned ratios of support that are based on individual needs and in accordance with governing rules and regulations.
- Provide person-centered supports which requires flexibility, creativity, and commitment.
- Facilitate participant involvement and engagement in purposeful activities and interactions while following established schedules of activity. Positively support and challenge participants to learn, maintain, and increase functional skills.
- Promote choice making, independence, socialization, behavior management, and communication.
- Assist participants in developing the necessary skills for personal success, including but not limited to, self-care, self-management, communication, and safety awareness.
- Model and ensure quality interaction by adhering to the organization's core competencies and core values.
- Ability to intervene in conflict and effectively communicate with participants.
- Know, understand, and uphold participants' rights, and immediately report any violations witnessed.
- Ensure the sanitation and overall cleanliness of participants' homes and work areas.
- Follow individual support plans (ISPs) and any other related individual support/treatment plans as prescribed. Document service delivery accurately, thoroughly, and in a timely manner.
- Write incident reports in a timely and professional manner.
- Report any medical concerns and safety hazards, including any incidents which may constitute a major unusual incident (MUI) immediately.

- Foster a positive and supportive relationship of partnership in all activities with the participants.
- Represent Bittersweet in a positive and professional manner whether on or off the property.
- Provide assistance to participants with personal hygiene as individually needed and prescribed, including assisting with bathroom responsibilities, ensuring participants complete shaving, brushing teeth, bathing/showering, shampooing, and dressing appropriately for the weather and recreational activities.
- Assist in the clean up of bodily fluids and biohazardous material as necessary.
- Safely and responsibly transport participants when necessary (if considered an acceptable driver by the insurance company).
- Assist and participate alongside participants in all daily living tasks and activities such as lawn mowing, shoveling, weeding, meal preparation, house cleaning, hiking, bike riding, and swimming.
- Provide coverage according to schedule which may include overtime, weekends, evenings, and overnight awake shifts; stay awake and alert at all times, unless assigned to a sleep shift while participants are sleeping.
- Report to your scheduled location on time, and if unable to report for work, or if there is a need to come in late, or leave early, follow the Bittersweet attendance policy.
- Attend all mandatory meetings, trainings, and in-services as required.

Skills:

- Possess and use empathy in all actions and interactions.
- Exceptional and adaptable oral communication as demonstrated through daily interaction with participants, family members, co-workers, and community members.
- Excellent written communication exemplified through daily documentation toward the completion of IEP goals, individuals' outcomes, and incident reports.
- Ability to respectfully negotiate with participants and present options when necessary.
- Ability to engage multiple participants in varied activities.
- Effectively work in teams with co-workers and participants.

- Actively demonstrate computer skills regarding email, time reporting, and client care applications.
- Ability to express patience in difficult situations.

Physical demands:

- Ability to responsibly operate a variety of household appliances to include but not limited to dishwasher, washing machine and dryer, microwave, stovetop, and vacuum.
- Ability to lift objects weighing up to 50 pounds.
- Ability to use crisis and emergency response training to physically support participants in times of behavioral, medical, and environmental emergencies.
- Position self to bend, crouch, run, and walk extensively (e.g., up to five miles at one time).
- Assist participants in bathing and hygiene activities.
- Perform any household labor needed.

Work environment:

- Consists of indoor, household, and outdoor farm environments.
- Exposure to cleaning supplies, blood, or other potentially infectious materials.
- Must be aware of and follow safety requirements and protocols.
- Maintain a positive attitude in times of crises and in stressful environments.

The mission of Bittersweet, Inc. is to positively impact the lives of individuals with autism and those whose lives they touch.

Personal Characteristics

Resumes specifying training and certification credentials do not always identify individuals who will be successful as a staff member at Bittersweet Farms. Certain personality and character traits are better indicators of the potential to become an exemplary direct support professional. Recruiting, selecting, training, and monitoring these individuals are multifaceted tasks and require time.

The job application and interview process, along with subsequent training and monitoring activities, focus not just on the information necessary to work with adults with autism, but also on how one exhibits the personal traits required of Bittersweet staff. Eight personal traits are considered to be high priority for Bittersweet staff.

1. Respect. Recognition of each person as a dynamic and multifaceted individual is imperative. Doing so includes respecting and responding to the immediate needs of the individual regardless of challenges and limitations. Staff must always consider and support the attainment of individual goals. (An example of how to plan for this is presented in Asa's schedule. See page 67.)
2. Empathy. A well-developed sense of empathy—as an alternative to sympathy—is a primary focus in the staff selection process. While one can teach a person about autism, it's almost impossible to teach them how to be empathetic.
3. Nurturing. Supporting and encouraging people with autism is central to working as a direct service professional at Bittersweet Farms. This is challenging and can be emotionally and physically stressful and tiring. It's essential for staff to avoid showing negative emotions when working with Bittersweet participants. Staff are encouraged to take advantage of the available stress management outlets available both inside and outside of their working environment.

DEALING WITH STRESSFUL SITUATIONS

Several years ago, identical twins enrolled at Bittersweet for day services. A major obstacle confronted staff. The young men refused to enter buildings. All efforts to encourage and support the two men did not seem to work. Inclement weather, darkness, and even the enticement of pleasant activities and mealtime had no effect on this behavior. Attempts to manage the situation physically resulted in aggression and an ensuing power struggle. It required a great deal of empathy on the part of staff to accept the distress these men were experiencing and to refrain from entering into any kind of power struggle.

Program supervisors identified staff who had the empathy and patience to work through the men's anxiety and redirect their obsessive behavior. The staff were rotated so that no one had the assignment every day. After a year, the men were going in and out of buildings with minimal anxiety. Fourteen years later, they are working with a job coach for eventual employment in the community. Now, when the initial problem behaviors occur, staff are able to deal with the participants' anxiety in a supportive way. This often involves redirection.

Redirection takes a negative situation and changes it into a positive one. Bittersweet staff use redirection to help residents rise above many of the anxieties and obsessive-compulsive tendencies that often come with the disability.

4. Professionalism. Embedded in the Bittersweet approach is the concept of customer service, which includes the ability of an organization to satisfy the needs and wants of its customers. Customer service also means treating others as you would like to be treated yourself. The most direct customers at Bittersweet are the residents. Staff are expected to integrate customer service into the culture at Bittersweet and consistently demonstrate a pro-customer stance in all interactions and exchanges.

5. Patience. The value and benefits of partnership are only realized if understood within a long-term context. Frustration sometimes occurs when anticipated results fail to materialize in a timely way. Patience and an appreciation of the process are essential components of the partnership model.

THE WAY PLANTS GROW

Healthy plants have roots that, though unseen, provide the structure and support needed to grow from seedling to mature plant. Consider what would occur if the plant was pulled up to check on how the roots were developing. Something similar occurs when working with Bittersweet participants. It might be tempting to abandon the structured supports because their effectiveness can't always be observed in the short term. If the structured supports are removed, however, any gains will wither and die. Patience and an appreciation of the developmental processes are required for real growth and change to take place.

6. Flexibility. Maintaining structure is undeniably important. However, a balance is required. The ability to adjust to a participant's mood, physical condition, or unforeseen disruptions without abandoning structure that can and should be maintained is vital.

7. Ability to negotiate. Negotiation is a powerful tool when used effectively. It expresses collaborative problem-solving and communicates a message of concern and support. Knowing when and how to encourage and confront, and when to back off in order to get as close as possible to the desired outcome without engaging in a power struggle is imperative. Staff must understand the distinct differences between negotiation and bribery. Negotiation is a means to collaborative problem-solving, whereas bribery is a plea bargain for compliance. Understanding the meaning or purpose behind the activity and appreciating its importance to the participant and greater community can be achieved through negotiation. It's circumvented through bribery.

NEGOTIATION OR BRIBERY: TWO SCENARIOS

Dave requests a second serving of cake. A staff member responds by saying, "No, there's only enough for each person to have one slice. You've already had your cake." Dave, who has significant difficulty in verbally expressing his unrelenting sweet tooth, reacts by pushing the staff member and grabbing the dessert of Ann who is sitting next to him. The staff member responds by physically removing Dave's newly "won prize." This leads to an escalating exchange of collective distress. Finally, the staff member "gives in" and finds another dessert for Dave. This seems to satisfy him.

In the second scenario when Dave requests another serving of cake, the staff member shows empathy by asking him if he is still hungry. She then explains that there is not enough cake for everyone to have a second piece. Her proactive approach indicates that the situation could distress his housemates. She suggests other options, such as having something else to eat or waiting to see if everyone wants his or her dessert. In the end, a few slices of cake remain after the meal. Dave and the staff member set aside a piece to be eaten later after the others have left the room.

The key to effective negotiation involves a keen understanding of the individual, his or her interests, compulsion, language, and concept comprehension. In this example, health factors—such as diabetes—may dictate the degree of viable options and must be considered in the negotiation process.

---

8. Ability to be a team player. Rigidity in performing only what is required by perceived assignments cannot and does not work in a true partnership approach. Working cooperatively with others and sharing information, workloads, and tasks are required of all Bittersweet staff. Each team member brings his or her own set of values, life experiences, perceptions, and skills to the situation. To function as a team, each member must contribute what he or she can and value the contributions of others.

Other Considerations

An important consideration underlying employment in a service industry such as Bittersweet Farms relates to the funds available to pay the people who provide direct support. Monetary rewards are undeniably lacking and do not correspond to the skills, responsibilities, and conditions required or involved. There are other rewards, however, such as an appreciation of the abilities of others, feelings of self-actualization, and the inner satisfaction that comes with a meaningful job well done. The ability to recognize the large victories in sometimes seemingly small successes brings a continual sense of self-worth not always available in other career paths.

One issue faced by agencies serving people with disabilities is high staff turnover. While this continues to be an issue for Bittersweet Farms, several measures are in place to address this concern. Strategies that are proving to be somewhat effective include flexible scheduling, regular team meetings, and ongoing staff support and training.

Staff training begins with a basic orientation and continues through a series of sessions related to specific components of the program. Orientation sessions include information about autism, components of the Bittersweet model (history, values, philosophy, framework), residents' rights, and prevention/intervention strategies. A central theme of the orientation relates to understanding the values and capabilities of those served and then seeking and building on these attributes to create quality of life. This philosophical understanding underlying Bittersweet's approach is a requisite for all potential employees before they are even scheduled to shadow or participate in a group. Integrated in all training topics are Bittersweet core values, including partnership development, respect, safety, and security. These principles apply to all relationships: staff/participant, staff/coworker, and administrator/employee relationships.

Mentoring is an integral part of the training process. This involves pairing a new employee with an experienced direct support professional who serves as a model and provides support to the trainee. The mentor and mentee continue working together for some time, at least until both are comfortable with the newly hired staff working on his or her own. One of the special challenges of newly hired staff is learning how to work in a partnership model. Once the training period is over, monitoring activities continue. These activities include periodic reviews and often involve opportunities for further professional development.

The comprehensive services provided at Bittersweet Farms depend on professionals with diverse expertise. These individuals may be employees or professionals under contract for specific services and may include medical professionals (physicians and nurses) and professionals providing various therapy services, such as speech/language, occupational, massage, and physical therapy. Specialists and counselors in behavior, diet/ nutrition, rehabilitation, social work, and vocational services are often included as members of the intervention team. Mental health professionals (psychologists/psychiatrists) are especially helpful. Bittersweet staff have also found that adjunct services, such as homeopathic and reiki/ therapy healing touch, can be effective.

While other services and therapies may be included, the interdisciplinary teams may consist of just a few members. What's critical for effective team functioning, however, is the designation of a team leader. The leader bears responsibility for gathering necessary information and bringing the team together for group meetings or in other prearranged systems for communicating. Team members differ in many ways, and each may bring to the meeting views not always accepted by others. The role of the team leader is to enable open dialogue and encourage respect for differing views and suggestions.

Bittersweet recognizes that staff attitude toward work, co-workers, and participants is an important component in maintaining a caring, creative, and effective workplace. The program emphasizes the importance of people caring about and supporting each other. This component of the program is critical for creating quality of life for the residents.

References

Durrani, H. (2014). Facilitating attachment in children with autism through art therapy: A case study. *Journal of Psychotherapy Integration, 24*(2), 99–108.

Gernsbacher, M. A. (2006). Toward a behavior of reciprocity. *Journal of Developmental Processes, 1*(1), 139–152.

Kaplan, R. S., & Steele, A. L. (2005). An analysis of music therapy program goals and outcomes for clients with diagnoses on the autism spectrum. *Journal of Music Therapy, XLII*(1), 2–19.

Karst, T. O., & Van Bourgondien, M. E. (1991). Adaptation and change in a residential farmstead community. In N. S. Giddan & J. J. Giddan (Eds.), *Autistic adults in bittersweet farms* (pp. 198–205). Binghamton, NY: The Haworth Press.

5   Aerobic and Active

Encouraging a person's engagement in structured, supported, and physical activity is fundamental to the Bittersweet philosophy. Aerobic and challenging endeavors are encouraged as teams work and play together. The active involvement of each person is a goal for all tasks and recreational activities. Active involvement develops functional learning at a person's ability level, enhances relationships and teamwork, and creates a community of support. Activities are also designed to provide sensory input for participants with significant sensory processing deficits.

Visitors to Bittersweet Farms often comment on the activity level they observe. Everyone, residents and staff, seem to be engaged in a variety of tasks or active recreational pursuits. Sitting, doing nothing, or passively watching TV is not part of the Bittersweet scene. Physical activity is a vital component of the Bittersweet approach, as it plays a critical role in the well-being of the residents. Physical activity such as walking, bending, stretching, and reaching is built into daily routines and activities.

SPRING CLEAN-UP

Residents benefit from digging, bending, pulling, and lifting, and all the physical exertion required in cleaning up the grounds around the farm. They also have the satisfaction of working in partnership with staff and enjoying the outcomes of improved grounds.

This chapter presents the background and rationale for the physical exercise component of the Bittersweet model. This component is considered critical to the success of the program. Daily schedules incorporate opportunities to promote physical effort. The types of recreational programs

DOI: 10.4324/9781003271048-6

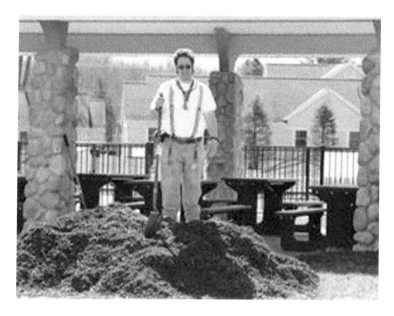

Figure 5.1 A Resident Enjoys the Heavy Work of Spreading Mulch in the Spring.

are numerous. Options for physical activity take into account the residents' age, interests, abilities, and disabilities. Along with a description of the physical activity program at Bittersweet, this chapter also provides information about how physical activities can be adapted or modified according to individual circumstances.

Background and Rationale

Bettye Ruth Kay maintained that vigorous exercise made a positive impact on the behavior, physical well-being, and attentiveness of her students. The work of Kijo Kitahara reinforced Kay's belief about the importance of exercise. Dr Kitahara (1984) developed a method of teaching that included vigorous physical exercise as a way to limit aggressive and self-stimulating or destructive behavior and to promote self-confidence and esteem. A comprehensive review of the literature on the benefits of physical activity for people with autistic spectrum disorder (ASD) conducted in 2010 identified 18 relevant studies. All 18 of the studies reported improvements in behavior, including reduced stereotypy, aggression, and self-injury. The most common behavioral improvement associated with increases in exercise was reduced stereo-typy or self-stimulatory behavior. This outcome was reported in 11 of the 18 studies (Lang et al., 2010).

Another reason why physical activity may reduce stereotypical behav-ior in people with ASD relates to feelings of anxiety and atypical responses to environmental stimuli. It is well documented that people with ASD are at greater risk for high levels of anxiety and depression than the gen-eral population (Marriage et al., 2009). In addition, individuals with ASD tend to have higher levels of sensitivity and over-arousal to environmen-tal stimuli which may cause anxiety. Physical activity is associated with a reduction in anxiety (Svensson et al., 2021).

Sensory Processing Disorders

All people interpret their world through sensory experiences. Most consider the following senses: seeing, hearing, touching, tasting, and smelling. Two additional senses that allow for environmental inter-pretation include proprioception (body position) and vestibular (bal-ance). People have proprioceptors which activate their proprioceptive sense within their joints and muscles. Experiences like deep pressure and heavy work activate the proprioceptive sense, allowing a person to know where his or her body is in relation to other objects and people. A person's vestibular sense is activated within his or her inner ear and controls balance.

Quality of life is supported when all the pieces of a person's sensory system work together in a collaborative way. Both neurological thresh-old and self-regulation play a role in achieving successful collaboration.

Neurological threshold is the amount of sensory input required to elicit a neurological response (Dunn, 2014). People with high thresholds require excessive input to reach their threshold, and generally have a limited ability to react to sensory information around them. People with low thresholds require little input and are typically distracted by all forms of sensory input. Self-regulation pertains to the way a person responds to sensory stimuli. Passive responders tend to let things happen before responding. Other people respond actively as related to their thresholds. Active responders attempt to regulate the amount and specific type of sensory input they receive (Dunn, 2014).

Bettye Ruth Kay developed her aerobic programing before much was known about sensory processing disorders. In 1983, her first residents did not have occupational therapy (OT) evaluations; and for the 20 residents studied in this program evaluation, OT reports and recommendations for specific exercise were not noted until the late 1990s. Yet, Bettye Ruth intuitively knew the value of vigorous exercise in helping participants become calm and less aggressive. Hiking in the woods promotes all the senses working together in a functional way and requires motor planning to get around trees!

WINTER HIKE

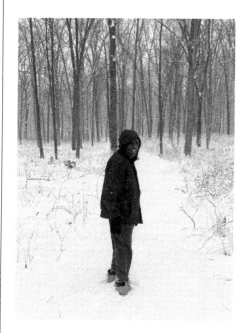

Figure 5.2 As Long as the Temperature Is Above Zero, Bittersweet Residents Go on Hikes.

Some research shows that sensory abnormalities are present in 94% of the ASD population (Crane et al., 2009). Yet, because of great variability in patterns of sensory processing impairments, individuals can experience very different, yet similarly severe sensory processing abnormalities. In adults with ASD, sensory processing abnormalities are relatively universal and can be very disabling (Gonthier et al., 2016).

A recent study demonstrated an association between sensory processing and aggressive behavior in adults with autism spectrum disorders (van den Boogert et al., 2021). Participants with greater sensory sensitivity had the highest risk of aggressive behavior.

The results of the program evaluation at Bittersweet indicate that at admission, 18 of the 20 residents studied had aggression, 9 of whom were severe. Twelve of the residents at admission exhibited self–injurious behaviors, six of whom were severe. The association of sensory processing and aggressive behaviors is important when planning interventions for residents with these presenting problems.

EXERCISE FOR BEHAVIOR MANAGEMENT

Ron's main problem when he entered Bittersweet Farms was aggressive outbursts. During the first few years, episodes of aggression occurred three to four times a day. Ron's aggressive outbursts were triggered by multiple situations; and the severity of the situation required staff working in partnership with him at all times. At one point, Ron began an exercise program of walking for 90 minute periods, three to four times a week. This program helped reduce his aggression and self-stimulatory behaviors. Over the years, other forms of aerobic activity were added to his work, therapeutic, and recreational programs. Ron responded well to the increased physical activities and, after several years in the program, participated in the Special Olympics. His incidents of aggressive behavior decreased dramatically—from three to four times per day when Ron first entered the program to currently about four to six per year.

Occupational therapy recommendations for residents profiled in the qualitative section of the program evaluation include specific activities that provide sensory stimulation in a meaningful context. Following are ten examples of such activities.

1. Shoveling snow with a small shovel. This activity provides proprioceptive as well as vestibular stimulation to balance the shovel, so the snow doesn't fall off. This activity also requires eye–hand coordination and provides tactile stimulation from wearing gloves and heavy winter clothing and boots.
2. Hiking in the snow and sledding. These activities require balance and provide vestibular stimulation.
3. Riding a bike on uneven terrain. This activity challenges a sense of balance and provides vestibular stimulation.

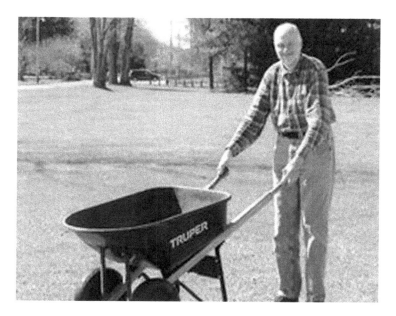

Figure 5.3 A Resident Enjoys Farm Work and Smiles while Pushing a Wheelbarrow.

4. Sweeping and mopping (filling a water bucket, adding soap, dumping dirty water).
5. Working in the barn (cleaning barn stalls, using the pump to get water, pouring the water into animal buckets, carrying buckets to the barn).
6. Mowing the lawn with an old-fashioned push mower.
7. Activities which require pushing and pulling.
8. Hiking in the woods.
9. Chopping wood, carrying logs, gathering sticks, pushing the wheelbarrow.
10. Ripping fabric and weaving.

Encouraging Physical Activity

ENCOURAGING PHYSICAL ACTIVITY

Why use weights and dumbbells?
Participating in a bell choir is so much more rewarding and it's fun!

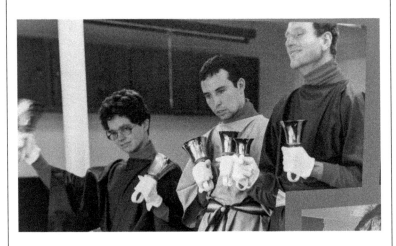

Figure 5.4 Residents Enjoy Performing in Bell Choir.

At Bittersweet, physical activities, such as hiking, bike riding, and roller-blading, are scheduled at the end of each workday. Residents are also free to use an outdoor quarter-mile track with ten stations for sensory stimulation at any time. The track is also used for field days and as a picnic area for families. The track is conveniently placed between living quarters to encourage its use by everyone. Residents are often seen walking the track during their free times. In addition, exercise is woven seamlessly into each participant's daily life in a calculated delivery of options and motivation. The Bittersweet philosophy incorporates exercise through the functional activities of farming, animal care, yard work, gardening, horticulture, and housework.

The physical layout of the buildings and the gardens has been planned to require greater physical activity. Buildings are spaced out to require walking a distance between them; and gardens are placed at far corners of the farm, so residents have a longer distance to carry produce. The compost heap is placed away from the gardens to again require a longer distance to carry weeds and debris. Bathrooms, located in a central location rather than in each building, also require walking between buildings.

While the general layout of the farm encourages walking, so do staff. Residents are often asked to take a message to someone who is on the other side of the farm, as a way to increase their physical activity levels. Requests and chores are planned with walking and exercise in mind.

Farming, animal care, horticulture, grounds maintenance, and clean-up are done the old fashion way to increase activity and to provide sensory input. There are no leaf blowers, large push brooms, electric saws, snow blowers, or other modern conveniences that shorten tasks and reduce heavy physical labor. Residents use hoes, rakes, and push carts as they work around the farm. They carry heavy loads of produce and work materials. The exercise they get while pulling weeds, planting, and repairing things around the farm is done within a meaningful context.

Bittersweet residents participate in many Special Olympic areas. Beth, shown in Figure 5.5, participated in the 2020 Special Olympics Ohio State Indoor Winter Games at Bowling Green University. She won gold in the women's 50 meter breaststroke, bronze in the women's 25 meter butterfly, and bronze in the women's 50 meter freestyle. Beth also earns medals each year in downhill skiing.

Many residents participate in the Special Olympics in swimming, tennis, basketball, and many other events. These activities promote aerobic exercise as well as sensory input. Other residents who do not participate enjoy being part of the pep club!

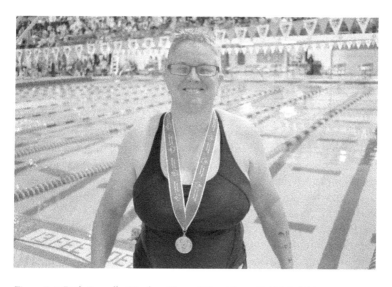

Figure 5.5 Beth Proudly Displays One of Her Many Gold Medals!

BUILDING ON SPECIAL INTERESTS

One female resident is not only limited because of a physical disability, but is also strongly turned off by any traditional aerobic activity. After the staff identified her strong interest in finding and collecting unique rocks and other "discoveries," they encouraged her to assist in weeding the gardens and outlying areas around the farm. While she would immediately dismiss the suggestion of a hike, she would gladly walk, bend, and pull weeds in hopes of finding a "treasure." By tapping into her individual interests, the staff were able to engage her in more physical activity than what she would otherwise be open to.

The physical activity program at Bittersweet is varied and woven into the very fabric of life on the farm. Residents benefit from the program by being more physically fit, gaining a better sense of body awareness, and experiencing pride in their accomplishments. Being physically active also contributes to quality of life by reducing stress and promoting inner tranquility (Kithara, 1984).

Physical Activity and Quality of Life

Being physically active can be an important contributor to quality of life. People with ASD, however, are less likely than people without disabilities to be physically active (Hillier et al., 2020) and more likely to lead a sedentary life. Approximately 50% of older individuals with intellectual disabilities, including ASD, living in community settings may be living dangerously sedentary lifestyles. Such individuals are more likely than individuals without developmental disabilities to experience related health problems, including cardiovascular disease, insulin resistance syndrome, and obesity. When exercise is increased for this population, however, improvements in physical health, intellectual functioning, perception, behavior, affect, and personality have all been reported (Lang et al., 2010).

The Bittersweet model emphasizes the importance of physical activity as a contributor to quality of life. The Bittersweet approach embeds exercise into meaningful activities related to work, relaxation, and recreation. The purpose associated with the activity increases the participant's motivation to engage in physical exercise. The Bittersweet model also values individualization. One reflection of this core value is demonstrated in the way physical exercise for an individual is planned around his or her preferences. Staff are aware that individualized physical activity plans tend to be not only more motivating, but also more beneficial in terms of outcomes. This approach is consistent with research findings. A comprehensive review of the literature found that individualized physical activity programs were more effective in promoting both motor and social functioning of people with ASD than group programs (Sowa & Meulenborek, 2012).

In addition to the physical benefits, engagement in meaningful physical activities also promotes several quality-of-life indicators, including self-confidence and pride in accomplishments.

References

Crane, L., Goddard, L., & Pring, L. (2009). Sensory processing in adults with autism spectrum disorders. *Autism*, *13*(3), 215–228.

Dunn, W. (2014). *Sensory profile 2 manual.* San Antonio, TX: Pearson.

Gonthier, C., Longuépée, L., & Bouvard, M. (2016). Sensory processing in low-functioning adults with autism spectrum disorder: Distinct sensory profiles and their relationships with behavioral dysfunction. *Journal of Autism and Developmental Disorders*, *46*(9), 3078–3089.

Hillier, A., Buckingham, A., & Schena, D. (2020). Physical activity among adults with autism: Participation, attitudes, and barriers. *Perceptual and Motor Skills*, *127*(5), 874–890.

Kitahara, K. (1984). *Daily life therapy: A method of educating autistic children. Record of actual Education at Musashino Higashi Gakuen School, Japan* (Vol. I). Boston, MA: Nimrod Press.

Lang, R., Koegel, L. K., Ashbaugh, K., Regester, A., Ence, W., & Smith, W. (2010). Physical exercise and individuals with autism spectrum disorders: A systematic review. *Research in Autism Spectrum Disorders*, *4*(4), 565–576.

Marriage, S., Wolverton, A., & Marriage, K. (2009). Autism spectrum disorder grown up: A chart review of adult functioning. *Journal of the Canadian Academy of Child and Adolescent Psychiatry*, *18*(4), 322–328.

Sowa, M., & Meulenborek, R. (2012). Effects of physical exercise on autism spectrum disorders: A meta-analysis. *Research in Autism Spectrum Disorder*, *6*(1), 46–57.

Svensson, M., Brundin, L., Erhardt, S., Hållmarker, U., James, S., & Deierborg, T. (2021). Physical activity is associated with lower long-term incidence of anxiety in a population-based, large-scale study. *Frontiers in Psychiatry*, *12*, 714014–714014.

van den Boogert, F., Sizoo, B., Spaan, P., Tolstra, S., Bouman, Y. H. A., Hoogendijk, W. J. G., & Roza, S. J. (2021). Sensory processing and aggressive behavior in adults with autism spectrum disorder. *Brain Sciences*, *11*(1), 95.

6   The Meaning Behind
Challenging Behaviors

Meaning and Motivation: The Communicative Intent

All behavior has a meaning and a purpose. How these are expressed is a fundamental concern in autism. Severe behaviors, such as screaming, aggression, self-injury, tantrums, and stereotypical/repetitive movements, are a way that people with autism typically communicate discomfort or distress. Unfortunately, these behaviors become the focus of many well-intended interventions, albeit inappropriate, that are imposed upon people with autism.

Interventions for challenging behaviors need to start with an understanding of what the individual seeks (meaning) and gets (motivation) from those behaviors. Motivation is "what" drives behavior; it is the "why" behaviors occur. From this vantage point, it is possible to develop intervention strategies by offering acceptable alternatives.

In her book, *Thinking in Pictures*, Temple Grandin (1995) noted that

> Some people with autism are like fearful animals in a world full of dangerous predators. They live in a constant state of fear, worrying about changes in routine and becoming upset if objects in their environment are moved. This fear of change may be an activation of ancient anti-predator mechanisms that are blocked or masked in most other people.

The cause of the individual's discomfort may be internal or external. Sensory or environmental disturbances which may seem minor sometimes lead to sudden outbursts. The most effective intervention begins with identifying the source of the stress. Once that has been identified, meaningful and lasting changes can be made.

Authoritative approaches are often used to address inappropriate behaviors. These approaches are usually ineffective, as they fail to reach

DOI: 10.4324/9781003271048-7

deeper than the surface level of the behavior. Authoritative approaches attempt to convey what is inappropriate, rude, or disrespectful and why. What's missing in this approach is an understanding that "behavior" is a form of communication and an emotional response. Focusing only on the response and not what triggered it sends the message that "you are not allowed to have these feelings." Such a message lacks understanding and empathy.

Consider the scenario of a resident screaming or yelling at his or her support person. The natural response might be to tell the resident, "You need to stop yelling," "We don't yell at other people," or "You need to calm down." Such statements often carry a tone of expectation and authority. It's natural for people who are already emotionally upset to become increasingly sensitive and vulnerable to additional distress. If, in response to their emotional distress, residents feel scolded, are told it's "wrong" to feel the way they do, and are given directions they believe are beyond their control, the situation will likely get worse.

One of the best responses to someone who is yelling at you is to empathically let the individual know that you want to help him or her but cannot understand what the individual is saying when he or she is yelling. Asking the individual politely and supportively to speak softer so that you can hear, understand, and help him or her extends a few important messages. First, you acknowledge that the person is upset and that you want to help. Second, you provide a function and rationale for what you are asking him or her to do. In this case, speaking softly isn't a matter of what "should" be done or what is "appropriate," but a matter of what is necessary in order to get the help and support the person wants. This approach also teaches individuals strategies they can use to become more self-reliant and less frustrated with others. This approach avoids placing the supporter in the middle of a moral battle. It places the individual at the center of the situation and encourages a greater sense of empowerment.

Most of us have probably had the experience of being upset and feeling that others weren't listening to us. What we probably wanted at that moment wasn't a resolution or a fix, but to be heard and have our concerns acknowledged. The same applies to the people with whom we work. When faced with challenging behaviors, our primary goal should be to foster a sense of trust. This involves letting the residents know that we're there to support them, not to be an enforcer keeping them from getting what they want.

Finding the reason for a resident's behavior can be complicated. The one message we can draw from challenging behaviors is that something is wrong. Discovering just what that "something" is requires the staff at Bittersweet to become "behavior detectives" in search of the "what" and "why" behind the behavior.

Good behavior detectives start by distinguishing between form and function. The form of behavior is the way a person behaves. It's the behavior itself. The function of behavior is the motivation behind what the person is doing. It's the "why" of the behavior. Identifying the form comes by way of observation. Labels—such as yelling, kicking, throwing, and hitting—are often used to describe what is observed (the form). There are two basic functions or reasons behind challenging behaviors: avoidance and wants. The individual exhibiting a challenging behavior is generally trying to avoid a situation or trying to get something he or she wants. To identify the function, a good behavior detective will look not just at the form of the behavior, but at what comes immediately before or after the behavior. This strategy is called a "functional assessment." The goal of this assessment process is to determine the relationship between events in the person's environment and the manifestation of the challenging behaviors.

At times, it's what *doesn't happen*—rather than what does happen—immediately before or after the challenging behavior that provides clues to the "why" or function of the behavior. Consider, for example, a staff member working in the garden with one of the residents. The task at the moment is digging carrots. After the process of removing a carrot from the ground is clearly demonstrated, the resident completes the task successfully several times. Smiles and "thumbs up" are exchanged each time a carrot is placed in a box. Later in the day, the two "gardeners" dig for potatoes. The resident, however, doesn't seem interested in the task. He tries several times to wander away from the garden. When redirected, he kicks the box of harvested potatoes and yells at the staff member. The potatoes that were harvested are now on the ground around the box. The staff member moves on to another potato plant, digs for the potatoes, and places them in the now empty box. She smiles and offers a "thumbs up." The resident stops yelling and starts digging for potatoes. He does a "thumbs up" for each potato he puts in the box.

The trigger of the behavior (yelling and kicking the box) was the resident's need for recognition or attention. The staff member was quick to recognize this. Once the attention was given, the resident became cooperative enough to, not only dig more potatoes, but also help pick up the potatoes he had knocked out of the box.

AFFIRMING THE PRESENT: A CALMING STRATEGY

Recently, a young man who lived in a distant city enrolled at Bittersweet. His family had ongoing involvement in his life. He was expected to come home for holidays and special occasions. Prior to going home, he seemed to become entangled in what can best be described as an "identity crisis." He fixated on past occurrences, inquiring about events and activities he'd previously experienced. He'd ask things such as "Do I ride bus 7 to school?" Then he instructed staff to say "No." His ending statements were always the same, "That was before" and "I am now a country gentleman farmer." Affirmation of his present reality became an obsession for him. He made repetitive drawings of images from his childhood. He continually called his parents with the same line of questions, always seeking assurance that his reality is not in the past, but in the present moment.

This young man exhibits some of the same behaviors seen in those suffering from posttraumatic stress disorder. Although we were unable to unlock the causes for his distress, we were able to support him in confirming his present reality. The anxiety he exhibited prior to visiting his family and city where he once lived was lessened by anticipating his need for affirmation of the present with calming reassurance until the visit was completed.

Challenging behaviors often associated with autism spectrum disorder (ASD) include repetitive movements of the body or objects, deliberate injury to the body, violent outbursts of rage, aggression, and non-compliance. These behaviors are often an attempt to communicate discomfort or stress. People with ASD may not have the ability to communicate needs and wants in appropriate ways. They use severe outward behaviors to express themselves. Such behaviors are their way of saying "Stop" or "I need help" (Grandin, 1995).

Triggers

Determining the cause, or causes, of challenging behaviors is critical to the effectiveness of an intervention. Identifying the cause determines the best way to respond. Bittersweet staff are trained to look for "triggers" (antecedents to the behavior) in the environment. Once recognized, triggers can be avoided or their effect minimized. Understanding and addressing the trigger of a challenging behavior lessen the potential for punitive or emotional reactions of persons working with people with ASD.

Many triggers are often overlooked, even though they are the most significant tool we have in understanding the individual and the behavior. Triggers could simply be one variable in the environment or a combination and accumulation of several variables. To identify the triggers, it's sometimes necessary to "rewind" back the minutes, hours, days, sometimes even the weeks building up to the incident or behavior in order to see the full array of potentially contributing factors. Table 6.1 provides examples of common triggers for people with ASD. As shown in Table 6.1, there are short-term and long-term triggers to consider.

As mentioned earlier, some triggers relate to events and situations which occur in the physical and social environment; other triggers occur due to what doesn't happen. Another important point relating to triggers is the understanding that triggers for challenging behaviors are often dissociated from the original stress. We might refer to these as "hidden triggers."

NOISE AS A TRIGGER

Larry is hyper-acoustic. At times, he'll put his hands over his ears to block out sound, even if the source of noise is no more than typical conversation. Noisier environments tend to trigger agitation and aggression. Staff members are aware of Larry's sensitivity to noise. If they notice any signs of agitation, they'll redirect him to a calmer setting. They also encourage him to use headphones in louder areas. When Larry becomes agitated or aggressive, staff approach him quietly and calmly. They always use low, soft voices when speaking to him.

The farmstead setting provides a variety of activities and options for individuals like Larry who have difficulty functioning in a noisy environment. Larry usually functions well with simple tasks in various areas around the farm, such as in the barn. When frustrated or sensitive to the noise, Larry can go outside and walk around to calm down.

Table 6.1 Common Triggers

	Examples/Descriptions
Short-Term Triggers	
Schedule changes	Even seemingly minor adjustments such as changes in activity, time, or personnel can trigger a negative response.
Ineffective communication	Words, gestures, or instructions not understood or misinterpreted may be causative factors for negative behavior.
Sensory response	Noise, temperature, color, smells, taste, textures, and proximity to others are potential sources of distress.
Lack of attention	Unmet cravings for attention can lead to disruptive behaviors.
Ritual disruption	Interrupting ritual obsessions, such as a need to follow a specific sequence, can create anxiety and result in negative outcomes.
Long-Term Triggers	
Change in support	Changes in staff or staff roles are a common cause of distress.
Loss of family members	Death, illness, or displacement of any person (or pet) who is key in the life of an individual can be a continuing source of distress.
Change of service or service location	Modification of a service, which may involve change in location, personnel, equipment, form of therapy, etc., may be disturbing.
Seasonal changes	Changes in the season or weather requiring different clothing and activities can be difficult for people with ASD.
Time changes	Time adjustments, including changes to and from daylight savings time and/or changes in the daily schedule, can be a cause of anxiety.
Medication changes	Changes in the types and/or dosages of medications can have a profound effect on behavior.
Upcoming events	Holidays, birthdays, special events, and any highly anticipated event may be a source of anxiety for people with ASD.

CHANGE AS A TRIGGER

George became a resident at Bittersweet Farms at the age of 19. His major challenges included anxiety, agitation, and obsessive-compulsive behaviors. His anxiety, short attention span, and agitation were limiting his ability to be happy and content with his surroundings. The farm setting has provided George with choices of varied tasks that are meaningful to his daily life. The setting also contributes to a sense of calmness, as it provides George with acres to walk or hike—activities which reduce his anxiety and stereotypic behavior. Yet, when things change, George has a tendency to get agitated.

George became agitated when a decorative peace pole was moved on the grounds during the construction of new housing. George became upset that it was in the wrong place; and different interventions failed. Eventually, the pole was removed to calm him down. The philosophy at Bittersweet is that the environment can be changed to accommodate the residents.

Behavior Modification: Emotional Response

Each resident has a crisis intervention plan with suggestions for ways to help him or her calm down and release excess energy if he or she becomes agitated. Most suggestions for calming down include preferred activities which incorporate some form of physical activity. Staff may take a resident for a walk on the track or through a trail in the woods. For all of us, movement and preferred activities have a way of calming us down and clearing our minds!

The approach used by typical behavior modification programs focuses on replacing undesirable behaviors with more desirable ones through positive or negative reinforcement. For those who "live in the moment" this treatment does not address the meaning (why) or motivation (what) for the behavior. It is, at best, a fragmented approach toward a desirable end. Behavior modification treatment ignores the communicative intent of the behavioral problems.

Emotions and feelings are a normal part of being human. Yet, when an individual has an emotional outburst, such as often seen in people with autism, the immediate response is to intervene. The intent is to stop the disruptive behavior quickly with little regard for the reason behind the behavior. In effect, the message sent is negative. The feelings and emotions that caused the outburst are not acceptable and the message given is that they are not important. The approach used for managing challenging behaviors at Bittersweet is based on the understanding that emotions and feelings are a normal part of being human. The first step in the intervention process involves identifying the function of the behavior—that is, understanding what the individual is trying to achieve. The ultimate goal is helping the individual learn more appropriate ways to achieve the outcomes he or she seeks.

Bittersweet combines some traditional components of behavior modification with a positive approach. The emphasis is on understanding that maladaptive behavior is either triggered and/or fueled by an unfulfilled emotional need.

To implement this approach, staff must be able to empathize with the individual's feelings or difficulties relating to the challenging behavior. Possibilities to consider include the need to ease fear, frustration, a loss of control, isolation, anxiety, anger, confusion, or a combination of emotions. The process of identifying "what's wrong" requires staff to have not just empathetic skills, but also an understanding of each of the participants. The Bittersweet partnership approach serves this function well. Staff—in their roles as teacher, partner, and guide—facilitate the discovery of ways that individuals can fulfill their needs in an appropriate manner. This process also promotes the development of the communication and problem-solving skills of the residents.

This positive behavioral approach might be described as "watering the flowers, not the weeds." The focus is on the "do's," not the "don'ts." This approach negates the power of the challenging behavior, allowing it to have no effect. Helping residents learn appropriate behaviors not only empowers them to have their needs met, but also promotes their sense of pride and self-respect.

Focusing on the positive in a behavior management program calls attention to the ultimate goal of the intervention—that is, improving the social skills, the communication skills, and the adaptive skills of the individual. The ultimate goal is about improving their quality of life, not making life easier for those around them.

Behavior management strategies using positive reinforcement and negative consequence as the basis for changing behaviors usually does not have a long-lasting effect on people with autism. One reason for this relates to the fact that people with ASD tend to have difficulty learning from experience. They may react to "old" memory as if it is occurring in the present. They may respond to "old" triggering events or anything that reminds them of such events. The concepts of "before" and "later" may not exist for them. The "now" may be their only reality. Whatever is in their immediate thought takes control of their actions. They may not be able to change their thoughts, see alternatives, consider another person's viewpoint, or shift their attention. Such issues need to be considered in the functional assessment of each individual.

When one perceives an external situation as threatening or fearful even in the absence of direct stressors, there is a "fight or flight" response. The anxiety may be caused by a strong aversion to external stimuli, internal stimuli, or social situations resulting in involuntary avoidance, diversion, fear, depression, retaliation responses, and defensive strategies. In autism, this can involve compulsive responses many view as inappropriate behaviors. Examining the "what" and "why" of behavior before reacting is the most important step in resolving behavior issues.

The "what" tends to be constant. The "why" does not disappear. The waxing and waning of distressing behaviors are common. Change takes a long time. Frustration takes its toll. It is not difficult to understand the urge to give up by saying, "tried that—it doesn't work." Autism doesn't respond to quick fixes, but the rewards that come through perseverance can be long-lasting for staff.

Related Issues

Challenging behaviors always occur in some type of context. Understanding related issues within these contexts can be helpful in identifying appropriate interventions. This section includes a discussion about six different issues to be considered in working with adults with ASD.

Sensory Issues

All of us exhibit repetitive behaviors at times. We might fidget, shift position, tap fingers or feet to help us concentrate on a task, calm anxieties, relax, feel more comfortable or in control. People with autism may exhibit repetitive behaviors which seem excessive or non-productive. Their stereotypical behaviors have been viewed by traditional behavioral theory as stigmatizing, distracting, unnecessary, and in some instances, as an act of defiance. Research (Prizant et al., 2006) suggests that these repetitive and apparently non-functional behaviors serve a self-regulatory and self-calming function in the same way fidgeting does in the general population. The classic characteristics of autism—such as hand-flapping, rocking, and other repetitive movements—serve the function of stimulating an under-registered nervous system or calming an over-registered system. From this perspective, stereotypical behavior serves an important function by helping to regulate emotions and the level of arousal.

Engaging in endless power struggles in order to help individuals curb or extinguish the distressing behavior is counterproductive, as it fails to understand the meaning behind the behavior. Yet, if the stereotypical behavior significantly impairs daily functioning, it may be necessary to substitute the stereotypical behavior with something more appropriate.

Many stereotypical behaviors are stigmatizing or disruptive to others in certain settings or situations. Finding and teaching more appropriate settings, times, or methods to obtain self-regulation is a necessity. Sensory processing strategies can be helpful in providing the needed self-regulation.

Sensory processing is a process that allows us to take in information through our senses, organize it, interpret its meaning, and respond accordingly to the environment. It also gives us the ability to filter out surrounding stimuli which may interfere with our daily functioning. People with ASD are often unable to regulate or modulate the input they receive through their senses. They may thus engage in stereotypical behaviors to help regulate their level of arousal.

Our basic senses are often listed as sight, hearing, touch, taste, and smell. These are the obvious senses. We have some hidden senses, as well. These include the vestibular sense and proprioceptive sense. These two hidden senses—along with the five basic senses—impact our ability to integrate the information we receive from the environment. The vestibular sense provides information about balance, movement, and gravity. It also impacts eye–hand coordination, that is, the way the eyes and hands work together. The proprioceptive system receives information from muscles, joints, and ligaments. This information helps us understand and control our body's movements and positions. The proprioceptive system plays a critical role in motor planning abilities. It helps us judge limb movements and positions, tells us how far to reach for an item, and indicates how much pressure is comfortable or uncomfortable on the body. The vestibular sense and the proprioceptive system work together as a foundation for purposeful movement.

As many as 80%–90% of individuals with ASD demonstrate sensory-related problem behaviors (Schaaf et al., 2010). These behaviors may have a sensory processing basis. The related condition is sometimes referred to as "sensory dysfunction" or "sensory processing dysfunction." People with this dysfunction find it difficult to analyze and respond appropriately to sensory input. Some research indicates that sensory dysfunction is one of the most significant factors limiting the ability of people with ASD to participate in home and community activities (Schaaf et al., 2010).

Some experts believe that many of the challenging behaviors commonly seen in people with ASD are due to sensory processing problems (Willis, 2006). Such problems may manifest as being over-sensitive (hypersensitivity) or under-sensitive (hyposensitivity) to sensory stimulation. With hypersensitivity (being overstimulated), a typical response is to block out the source of stimulation. Manifestations of such a response include covering one's eyes when lights are too bright or covering one's ears when the environment is too noisy. Other manifestations of hypersensitivity include sniffing the air or other people, being very sensitive to textures, and not liking to move. With hyposensitivity (being under-stimulated), a typical response is to seek sensory stimulation. Manifestations of this include staring at flickering fluorescent lights, speaking and/or singing loudly, seeking out items that make loud noises (e.g., whistles), rocking back and forth, spinning, and licking non-food objects. Being under-sensitive places individuals at greater risk for getting hurt. People who are hyposensitive might pick up hot objects or walk into traffic.

The nature-filled environment at Bittersweet gives residents many opportunities for multisensory experiences, such as hiking in the woods, pushing an old-fashioned lawn mower, or chopping wood and hauling it in a wheelbarrow. Some research indicates that sensory-rich environments may contribute to calm behavior and/or self-regulation in individuals with ASD (Scartazza et al., 2020). In addition to exposure to the nature-rich physical environment, specific sensory activities scheduled throughout the day provide residents with sensory experiences. Some such activities incorporate specific sensory processing strategies in a positive and consistent manner. Sensory supports, such as weighted vests or backpacks, are also used, as needed. Care is taken to avoid placing residents in situations where they will be over stimulated. For example, natural light (versus florescent light) is used when possible. Noisy tools, such as electric saws and leaf blowers, are not used; instead, wood is cut with a two-man saw and leaves are raked by hand. The farm setting is very calming, and if a resident is upset, interventions include walking around the farm or hiking in the woods.

The resident shown in Figure 6.1 receives needed sensory input by ripping cloth into strips and weaving them into rugs. Part of sensory processing involves being able to use the sensory systems together. Weaving involves using the visual and tactile systems together. Weaving also improves fine-motor coordination (something many people with autism have difficulties with) and visual-motor integration. The repetitive movement is also very calming.

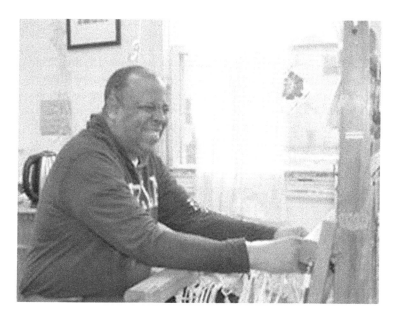

Figure 6.1 A Resident Enjoys the Repetitive Movement of Weaving On a Loom.

Environmental Issues

The inability to generalize information and to learn from one context to another is inherent in autism. Change is particularly difficult. Unexpected changes in the physical and social environment—such as changes in routines, locations, or staff—are likely to cause anxiety and distress. Something as seemingly insignificant as the beginning and end of daylight savings time is particularly difficult for many Bittersweet participants. The emotional response to change for people with ASD often takes the form of confusion, frustration, anxiety, and anger. People with ASD are less able to understand that one change of context does not necessarily negate all other variables within the routine. Bittersweet staff understand this concern and provide support for the residents by preparing them in advance for anticipated changes. Social stories, schedules, and visual supports are helpful in this process.

Many changes, however, cannot be foreseen. Staff respond to unexpected changes by providing an immediate explanation of why the change is occurring. They calmly describe the change and reassure the residents that the change is temporary and that the routine will resume.

THE FLAT TIRE

It started out like a routine shopping trip. Tim and Jenny, both non-verbal residents, were well prepared and looking forward to their trip to a grocery store. Jon, a long-time support staff member, knew both residents very well. Shortly after the journey began, Jon felt a jolt that signaled a flat tire. He slowly pulled to the side of the road and, before opening the door of the vehicle, calmly signed and gestured the problem. "… flat tire." He indicated he could fix the tire and they would continue to the store. Only then did he leave the vehicle. Both residents indicated they wanted to see. Jon continued to sign and gesture through every step of the process. In a short time, the new tire was in place and the shopping trip resumed as scheduled.

PREPARING FOR CHANGE

Periodic changes in staff assignments at Bittersweet are necessary. Helping residents feel comfortable with even subtle change can be a daunting task. A well thought out and planned course of action is needed to alleviate anxiety and help residents adapt to and cope with inevitable change.

The first step in this process is to frequently review with the residents a calendar with schedules. Incoming staff are then introduced by having them overlap with the outgoing staff, always maintaining and calling attention to the structural integrity of the process. This process gives the staff the opportunity to explain not only the changes, but also the "why" behind them.

Physical Issues

Autism is a neurological and developmental disorder that can impact the entire body as a result of communication deficits. Some physical ailments may be small and/or not visually evident, yet painful. A middle ear infection or a build-up of wax, for example, may cause discomfort in the ear. A person with autism may respond with ear slapping because they cannot directly communicate. Due to the communication deficits of the residents at Bittersweet, staff need to have a working knowledge of each individual's normal range of affect and behavior so that they can detect when something is amiss.

Social Issues

For residents, living and working with others is not always easy, especially when those you work with need individualized services and supports and are prone to episodic distress with its varying manifestations. Often, stress expressed by one individual can cause a chain reaction. This makes it imperative for staff at Bittersweet to be aware of the social issues between residents and work toward effective mediation of conflicts as they arise.

Giving time, attention, and support to those who may be less involved in a situation may keep them calm.

REDUCING CONFLICT IN GROUPS

Paul often responds with loud crying when he gets upset. He's been known to cry for up to three hours at a time. While this behavior reflects Paul's distress, the loud crying also distresses and disturbs people around him. At times, other residents will begin to cry or show other signs of anxiety. An appropriate staff response requires knowing each individual. While some residents are able to use words to express their concern, others can't.

In dealing with the stressful situation at hand, staff have two options: remove Paul from the others; remove others from Paul. A staff member might invite Paul to go for a walk in the woods or suggest that he goes along to care for the animals. A change in location and focusing on a preferred activity are often helpful. The other alternative is to remove others from where Paul is crying. This might involve a group walk in the woods or around the track.

Quality-of-Life Issues

The professional literature and guidelines for services typically call for "community integration" or "social inclusion" as an integral component of quality of life for individuals with disabilities. Yet, certain emotional and behavioral characteristics of people with autism indicate that such integration (as typically defined) may not always be workable or desirable. Many people with autism are challenged by severe forms of anxiety. Being around other people—especially when there are high expectations for socially appropriate behaviors—can intensify the anxiety and lead to aggressive behaviors.

The Bittersweet model recognizes the importance of community integration and social inclusion to quality of life but also realizes the necessity of individualizing the process. Adults with autism who come to Bittersweet do so because life elsewhere wasn't working for them. Many come with severe emotional and behavioral problems, often expressed through aggressive and violent actions, such as hitting people and throwing objects. This was the case with Larry whose main problem when he entered Bittersweet was aggression.

Larry moved to Bittersweet Farms at the age of 18. Test results indicated that he had an IQ of about 33. Larry's self-care skills (toileting and eating) and verbal language skills were very limited. His receptive language skills were somewhat better, and he was able to follow two-step directions. Larry's severely aggressive behaviors when he first came to Bittersweet were disruptive and costly. At one point, he picked up a bike and threw it at a car. On a number of occasions, he plugged toilets and flooded the bathroom floor.

Larry was placed in the farmworker program at Bittersweet Farms where he engaged in a combination of routine barn tasks and seasonal outdoor activities, such as gardening, orchard, and woodland work. He was also included in physically active recreational exercises, such as hiking, biking, and swimming. To increase his awareness of and interactions with others, Larry was also included in community activities, such as going to restaurants and the movies.

Even after several years of programming at Bittersweet, Larry was still resistant to being in his vocational placement. He would sit on the ground and rock for hours at a time, refusing to participate in any activity. He would often scream himself hoarse, which was disruptive to other participants. A number of behavioral intervention strategies were unsuccessful. This was attributed to Larry's low IQ and his inability to generalize learning, a common characteristic of people with autism. Vocationally, Larry continued to be inflexible in his ability to transfer from one area to another.

Staff allowed Larry to choose work which met his need for sensory input. He loves cutting wood rather than trying to sand a piece of wood evenly. A sanding project for him typically ends up with a groove in one spot; but Larry can cut wood for hours. At one point, Larry worked in a sheltered workshop doing repetitive tasks. He did this for over 15 years.

Once that work ended, Larry's aggressive behaviors escalated. When Larry is physically aggressive, staff are encouraged to back away and give Larry space. Staff make a point of not emotionally or negatively reacting to his aggression. They will block kicks, hits, or thrown objects with crossed arms and open palms or use a soft cushion or blocking pad to absorb any force.

Behavioral interventions include helping Larry verbalize his anger through appropriate words and volume. They also provide a quiet environment which seems to help Larry relax. At times, staff will ask Larry to take a walk and reassure him that he is in a safe place. Staff are encouraged to talk with him about his interest in Star Wars and Batman, give him compliments, and explain reasons behind requests. They also review behavioral and task-related expectations.

Larry now enjoys magazines/catalogues, shooting basketball hoops, playing catch, dining out, watching movies, and being engaged in hands-on tasks. He enjoys walking around the track and does so almost every day. While he doesn't enjoy participating in sports, Larry enjoys going to baseball games. Larry still needs continuous supervision at Bittersweet Farms, but may spend some time alone. Because Larry's behavior has improved, he participates in community activities and averages about six per month, mostly for shopping, swimming, going to church and library, and walking in various parks. Larry also attends summer camping trips and fairs.

References

Grandin, T. (1995). *Thinking in pictures: And other reports from my life with autism*. New York: Random House.

Prizant, B., Wetherby, A., Rubin, E., Laurent, A., & Rydell, P. (2006). *The SCERTS® model: A comprehensive educational approach for children with autism spectrum disorders*. Baltimore, MD: Paul H. Brookes.

Scartazza, A., Mancini, M. L., Proietti, S., Moscatello, S., Mattioni, C., Costantini, F., … Massacci, A. (2020). Caring local biodiversity in a healing garden: Therapeutic benefits in young subjects with autism. *Urban Forestry and Urban Greening, 47,* 126511. https://doi.org/10.1016/j.ufug.2019.126511.

Schaaf, R. C., Toth-Cohen, S., Johnson, S. L., Outten, G., & Benevides, T. W. (2010). The everyday routines of families of children with autism: Examining the impact of sensory processing difficulties on the family. *Autism*, 15(3), 373–389.

Willis, C. (2006). *Teaching young children with autism spectrum disorder*. Lewisville, NC: Gryphon House.

7 Quality of Life at Bittersweet

Discussions about autism spectrum disorder (ASD) often highlight deficiencies; and interventions for people with ASD tend to focus on minimizing deficits. Bittersweet takes a different approach by focusing on the strengths, capabilities, and interests of individuals with ASD. At Bittersweet Farms, people with ASD are viewed as being neurodiverse rather than deficient. This more positive perspective is strongly supported in the literature (Masataka, 2017; Robertson, 2010). While the deficit model portrays people with autism as broken in need of fixing, the neurodiversity perspective portrays the condition as a form of human diversity with associated strengths and difficulties (Robertson, 2010). The entire program at Bittersweet revolves around this more positive approach. The ultimate goal of the Bittersweet model is to provide a supportive environment where each individual can enjoy quality of life (QOL). This chapter highlights ways in which the Bittersweet model integrates an emphasis on quality of life with the neurodiverse perspective on adults with ASD.

Quality-of-Life Domains

Quality of life is sometimes defined and measured in relation to eight domains: interpersonal relations, social inclusion, personal development, physical well-being, self-determination, material well-being, emotional well-being, and human and legal rights (Schalock, 2004). The Bittersweet model considers each of these domains at the individual, organizational, and systems levels of support. With a person-centered approach, however, the emphasis is on the achievement of valued personal outcomes rather than meeting objective criteria relating to each of the QOL domains. Valued personal QOL outcomes are defined by the aspirations of the individual, which may not always be reflected in community indicators of QOL.

DOI: 10.4324/9781003271048-8

While there are both subjective and objective components to each of the QOL indicators, evaluation of quality is subjective. Most of the literature on QOL, however, is consistent in identifying self-determination, support, purpose in life, and a sense of belonging as key components in subjective QOL (Schalock, 2004). Some research focusing specifically on QOL for adults with ASD suggests that "good outcomes" for this population include such markers as working in valued jobs, participating in family and community activities, learning to make choices, and generally feeling happy (Bishop-Fitzpatrick et al.,

Table 7.1 Quality-of-Life Domains

Domain	Common Indicators	Bittersweet Supports
Emotional well-being	Contentment, self-concept, minimal stress, spirituality, happiness, safety	Predictability, consistency, person-first planning
Interpersonal relations	Social interactions, affection, family, friendships, support, personal relationships	Partnership, social activities
Material well-being	Shelter, employment, ownership, possessions	Meaningful work (valued jobs), purposeful activities, secure living arrangements
Personal development	Education, skills, personal competence, performance, advancement	Apprenticeship model, promoting competence, productivity, purposeful activity
Physical well-being	Health, nutrition, recreation, mobility, healthcare	Physical activity for daily living and recreation, choices
Self-determination	Autonomy, choices, self-direction, personal goals/values	Personal choices, varied multileveled activities, symbolic communication systems
Social inclusion	Community activities/integration, community roles, social support, acceptance, status	Volunteer opportunities, community outings, group activities, social belonging, meaningful engagement
Rights	Dignity, respect, privacy, access, ownership	Individualization

2016). As Table 7.1 indicates, each of these areas is addressed in the Bittersweet model.

Issues and Interventions

The growing population of adults with ASD has ignited increased interest and research in desired outcomes and quality of life for this population (Bishop-Fitzpatrick et al., 2016). Current research indicates that most adults with ASD do not achieve the conventional markers of adulthood (i.e., becoming self-supporting, living independently, and developing a network of friends) and that their QOL is deemed to be generally poor (Bishop-Fitzpatrick et al., 2016).

While adults with ASD face challenges to quality of life, they also have certain gifts which, in a supportive environment, can help them attain success in each of the QOL domains. The following discussion addresses some of these challenges and ways in which the Bittersweet model supports adults with ASD experience QOL in each of the eight domains.

Emotional Well-Being

Adults with ASD tend to experience different forms and much higher rates of anxiety than the general population (Robertson, 2010). The different forms include social anxiety, generalized anxiety, separation anxiety, and panic disorder (Gillot & Standen, 2007). Anxiety, in any form, is a major obstacle to emotional well-being.

The Bittersweet approach to addressing anxiety includes minimizing stress through predictability, consistency, and control. Various calming measures are also used, such as speaking in a soft voice, providing places to retreat, and capitalizing on residents' interests and abilities. The story of Jon, one of the residents at Bittersweet, attests to the effectiveness of the Bittersweet model in promoting emotional well-being.

After participating in the Bittersweet program for a number of years, Jon described his life as "going very good." This description was dramatically different from what the staff observed when Jon first came to Bittersweet. Jon was often aggressive, and if staff intervened, he would become violent. He also demonstrated inappropriate sexual behaviors and obsessions, destroyed property, and took money and other objects from people around him. His interaction with staff was limited to his wants and needs; and most of his language was ritualistic. Jon was also severely withdrawn and anxious.

Incorporating Jon into the structure of the farm and establishing relationships with the staff through partnership activities were the first steps in his intervention. Jon responded well to the structure of the farm and the constant supervision. Initially, Jon participated in the horticulture department at the prevocational level, learning farm life skills. Over time, the daily schedule of work in partnership with staff helped reduce his anxiety as he learned new skills and became more focused on activities. His communication skills also improved through his interactions with staff.

In addition to physically demanding farm work, Jon was also scheduled for vigorous exercise three times a week. The farm work required Jon to lift, carry items, and walk. These physical activities helped reduce his anxiety by providing him with proprioceptive input. Behavior plans were developed for Jon to help eliminate his inappropriate sexual behavior. Periods of time without demonstrating these behaviors earned Jon extra phone calls and visits with his family. After three months, there was a noticeable decrease in sexual behaviors. An annual review indicated that these behaviors were reduced to three in the past three months, down from 15 incidents per month the previous year. Several years later, there were no incidents of sexual behavior.

Once the inappropriate sexual behaviors were eliminated, Jon was able to become more integrated into the Bittersweet community. He participated in activities and jobs in which he excelled. Jon is now more content and less anxious. Through productive work, he now demonstrates a sense of self-worth. He enjoys the status of being an expert in using the rototiller, for example. Jon enjoys leisure activities, such as swimming at the Y and hiking every day. Jon has also participated in the Special Olympics.

In describing his life as "going very good," Jon highlighted some of the options and choices available to him. He listens to music, rides a bike, and works in several areas around the farm, including the art room, workshop, kitchen, and horticulture areas.

Interpersonal Relations

Growth in interpersonal relations involves developing friendships and other social relationships. People with ASD face major challenges throughout this process, as difficulties in language, communication, and social interaction are typical characteristics of the condition. While some resources have been developed for promoting social relationships for people with ASD, most such resources focus specifically on children and youth with ASD. There exists a profound lack of resources for helping adults with ASD navigate social relationships (Robertson, 2010).

Online social interactions seem to help some adults with ASD develop social relationships. Online-only relationships, however, do not allow for such shared activities as participating in sports, attending concerts and festivals, and eating together.

The partnership approach—which is integral to the Bittersweet model—promotes interpersonal relations through ongoing mutual support and collaborative side-by-side job sharing. Residents experience the "give and take" of social interactions as they partner with staff in the daily activities of the farm. The completion of activities, such as harvesting produce or mowing the lawn, is often celebrated with "high-fives," "thumbs-up," and shared smiles.

Susan, one of the residents mentioned in Chapter 3, made remarkable progress in the area of interpersonal relations after she moved to Bittersweet Farms. This was facilitated by the partnership aspect of the Bittersweet model. When Susan first came to Bittersweet, she needed one-on-one supervision, and all tasks were done in an interactive partnership with staff. Over time, Susan was able to interact socially with her caretakers and be responsive to other residents. The partnership activities also helped Susan improve her communication skills, including the use of sign language. While she knew some sign language when she first came to Bittersweet, she never used it until working with staff in a partnership arrangement. Two years after her admission to Bittersweet, Susan was forming significant attachments with others, primarily with direct care staff. In an effort to promote such attachments, staff working with Susan were kept as consistent as possible.

Material Well-Being

Work status plays a major role in material well-being. For adults with ASD, securing and sustaining meaningful work tend to be major challenges. Rates of underemployment and unemployment are much higher for adults with ASD than for people without ASD (Robertson, 2010). Underemployment refers to an employment status where a person's work (or job) underutilizes his or her skills and talents. Unemployment refers to an employment status where a person is without a job for an extended period of time.

Major job-related obstacles for people with autism include (a) acclimating to new procedures and routines, (b) meeting the social and communication demands of the work situation, (c) handling the sensory demands of the work environment, (d) engaging in goal-oriented and reflexive thinking, and (e) handling negative attitudes and stigma associated with autism (Robertson, 2010).

Material well-being for many adults with autism is also compromised by the lack of compatible living options. A large percentage of adults with ASD continue to live with their parents, who are often unable to provide the necessary support.

Bittersweet Farms addresses both the employment and living concerns related to the material well-being quality-of-life domain. Everyone at the farm is involved in meaningful work. All work-related responsibilities reflect the abilities and interests of the individual residents. Living arrangements, which provide security and safety, are also designed around the needs and abilities of the residents. Some Bittersweet residents need 24-hour supervision to maintain their safety; others function well in a co-op living situation.

MATERIAL WELL-BEING

Ben moved to Bittersweet Farms at the age of 19 because his parents were no longer able to provide the support and structure Ben needed to function at home. He was often at risk because of his wandering and inattention to traffic and machinery. Without a structured residential placement, Ben could have been injured and/or required police intervention as a result of his wandering into other people's homes.

The primary issue for staff when Ben first came to Bittersweet was maintaining his safety. Ben displays an obsession for wandering off the grounds and attempting to consume unsafe foods or other items. At times, Ben would leave the property and be found in a neighbor's house eating from his or her refrigerator. His favorites seemed to be cookies and pop. Initially, to maintain Ben's safety, Bittersweet Farms provided 24-hour supervision. Currently, a staff member keeps him in sight at all times and follows him if he attempts to run off. A door alarm is used during the night, so that a staff member is alerted if Ben wanders out of the house. Ben's episodes of running off did not appear to be triggered by anxiety or agitation but simply by opportunity. He would wait until staff were distracted and run off.

Over the years, various methods have been used and investigated, including using a motion alarm, researching personal location devices, and finally installing a front gate and fence. Finding a way to contain Ben was critical because without success, Ben would have had to be placed in an institution. At Bittersweet, Ben was moved from a 15-bed home to an 8-bed home to provide more supervision. He was given one-on-one supervision, which had many positive benefits in addition to keeping him from running off. The staff engaged Ben in more physical activity and gave him more positive attention. Over time, Ben's communication improved, and he was better able to express his needs. Occasionally, Ben will still run from a work setting, but his wandering behaviors have decreased significantly as a result of the interventions used by Bittersweet staff.

Personal Development

One of the universal capabilities shared by all humans is the "capability to develop" (Chawla, 2015; Nussbaum, 2011). Optimal development, however, doesn't just happen. A supportive environment is required for optimal development to occur.

The Bittersweet model recognizes that the components of what constitutes a supportive environment can differ from person to person. Individualization plays a key role in making Bittersweet Farms a supportive environment for all the participants. The process includes getting to know the strengths, needs, interests, goals, and concerns of each individual participant and then creating a social and physical environment that reflects the individuality of each participant. The entire program is built around the development of competence and the experience of success.

The apprenticeship approach used at Bittersweet Farms works well for promoting personal development. This approach allows residents to engage in work that is of interest to them and at their own ability level. Because the apprenticeship model involves working in partnership with staff, participants are given the time and support they need to learn new skills. The effectiveness of this approach is clearly demonstrated in the case of Gus.

Gus had a limited quality of life when he arrived at Bittersweet. His unpredictable and sudden hitting made it difficult to take him out in public. His independence was limited, and he had no specific skills. He had difficulty with self-care skills and limited interaction with others.

Gus' long-term goal was to eliminate aggression and to develop self-control. The staff used a number of different intervention techniques to help Gus achieve his goal. They continue using these techniques today.

The staff inform Gus of the schedule each day and evening at the beginning of each shift. They give explanations and suggestions rather than "orders." Corrections are always given in an indirect manner. Gus is encouraged to verbalize his feelings and frustrations. If Gus appears anxious, staff try to find out what is bothering him and help him problem solve. If Gus wants to run to calm himself, the staff encourage him to first complete a portion of the task in which he was involved so that running does not become an avoidance technique.

At Bittersweet, Gus learned to be productive through years in horticulture therapy, gardening, and crafting with a good teacher and therapist. Soon after the art program started, Gus found his home as a creative artist. His paintings are in demand and typically sell first at art shows. Gus is no longer socially isolated and now has skills in several areas that give him purpose and enjoyment. He enjoys many community activities, such as shopping, movies, art exhibits, and eating out.

The farmstead model provided the structured programming Gus needed to reduce his anxiety and to develop prevocational skills. Purposeful activities, such as working with animals, helped Gus to focus his attention on something outside of himself. All the activities are done in partnership with staff, which has allowed Gus to develop relationships and increase his communication skills. When Gus first came to Bittersweet, he needed to run to calm himself when agitated. He would often run for an hour or more in the front yard. Gus has profited from the active recreational program of hiking, sports, and the Special Olympics. The farm setting, with long distances to walk and physical chores to complete while taking care of animals and maintaining the property, has helped Gus reduce his anxiety. During his free time, Gus walks miles around the track each day. As Gus became more independent and his self-help skills increased, he moved into co-op housing with five other male participants. In this co-op setting, Gus participates in cooking and cleaning. He enjoys more independence and can tolerate his housemates.

Physical Well-Being

One of the concerns about quality of life for adults with autism is the lack of supportive recreational and physical activity programs (Robertson, 2010). This concern relates to the fact that many organized recreational programs include high social demands, which people with autism have a hard time meeting. This concern may also relate to a common misunderstanding that people with autism have a strong aversion to participating in social recreational opportunities. This misunderstanding may deter community organizations and groups from modifying their recreational programs to accommodate the needs of people with autism. Lack of opportunity may also lead adults with autism to focus their pastimes exclusively on solo hobbies despite potential interests in participating in social recreational programs (Robertson, 2010).

Incorporating physical activity in daily life is an essential component of the Bittersweet model. While vigorous physical activity is appreciated as a strategy for reducing aggressive and self-stimulating behaviors, it's also recognized as a way to promote self-confidence and self-esteem. Additionally, the physical activity program at Bittersweet allows participants to enjoy the health benefits and recreational aspects of being physically active.

PHYSICAL WELL-BEING

Ian attended special education classes through high school and had a positive attitude toward his teachers and school. Many of his behaviors were consistent with his diagnosis of autism. He demonstrated a lack of awareness of others and had severely impaired ability to make peer friendships. Ian was generally withdrawn, sitting for long periods of time staring. His main problem when he moved to Bittersweet was his tendency to withdraw. He had extreme difficulty remaining on task without continual staff supervision, including tasks he knew how to perform. There seemed to be no clear pattern or cause for his withdrawal, but this behavior interfered with Ian's ability to be independent, productive, and integrated into the Bittersweet community. Consequently, Ian had poor relationships with his peers and difficulty focusing on all aspects of his daily life.

An intervention plan developed for Ian at Bittersweet included participation in vigorous activities, which required attention in order to participate, such as tennis, baseball, and volleyball. Vocationally, Ian was placed in horticulture and animal care, both requiring large motor skills and designed to help him focus his attention. This treatment plan was successful for Ian. He likes living on the farm and enjoys groundskeeping and working in the horticultural program. Ian loves being physically active and participated in the Special Olympics in tennis. He flew to the 2000 Nationals with a group of other Special Olympians. He enjoys the recognition he receives for excelling in sports, especially for his awards in tennis.

Ian is now less withdrawn, has developed friendships, displays improved interactive skills, and demonstrates a sense of responsibility and motivation. The Bittersweet model, with its emphasis on community interaction, partnership, structure, and aerobic activity, has allowed Ian to transform over the years to where he can now enjoy quality of life.

Self-Determination

Individuals are self-determined if they act in a self-directed manner and their behaviors are self-regulated. Choice-making, decision-making, problem-solving, and goal setting all play a role in self-determination. Related research indicates that individuals with higher levels of self-determination also report higher perceptions of life satisfaction (Strnadova & Evans, 2012; White et al., 2018). A major barrier to the achievement of self-determination for people with autism is the mistaken assumption that self-determination is not attainable for many people on the autism spectrum. Some people may also have mistaken ideas about how people with disabilities rate the importance of self-determination in their lives. One study involving almost 800 people with intellectual disabilities, almost 500 family members of a person with disabilities, and over 770 professionals working with people with disabilities found that self-determination was rated significantly higher by the people with disabilities than did the professionals and family members. In fact, of all the quality-of-life core dimensions, professionals and family members rated self-determination as the lowest in importance to them (White et al., 2018).

The Bittersweet approach is based on a different belief system, one that incorporates the idea that everyone has the ability to exercise self-determination in some form. Bittersweet, therefore, promotes empowerment, choice, and independence. Bittersweet staff are aware of the importance of communication for self-determination and use various strategies and devices to help residents communicate their needs, feelings, and preferences. People without a working means of communicating are at a huge disadvantage in exercising self-determination (Robertson, 2010).

Many people with autism have serious expressive language disabilities which may be due to dyspraxia, generalized and social anxiety, and other conditions. While the use of augmentative and alternative communication (AAC) systems and other technologies has proven effective in enhancing the quality of life for people with various forms of disabilities, a large percentage of language-limited people with autism do not have adequate access to AAC or other language support systems that are compatible with their individual strengths and difficulties (Robertson, 2010). It's different at Bittersweet, where various strategies and devices are used to help residents communicate their needs, feelings, and preferences. Some of these strategies and devices are discussed in Chapter 3, and their effectiveness is illustrated in the following story about Oscar.

SELF-DETERMINATION: OSCAR'S STORY

Oscar was placed at Bittersweet Farms because his mother wanted a program that was structured and could provide Oscar with productive activities. Oscar was diagnosed as autistic as a child and was in special education classes in both private and public school settings. He was one of the students in Bettye Ruth Kay's class in Libbey High School.

In addition to autism, Oscar has obsessive-compulsive disorder. He functions in the mild range of mental retardation. A speech therapy evaluation at Oscar's admission to Bittersweet indicated limited language skills, with both expressive and receptive scores at about the five-year-old level of functioning. Oscar was approximately 25 at the time. Intervention goals for Oscar included becoming as independent as possible.

Oscar exhibited extreme ritualistic behaviors when he first came to Bittersweet. Interruptions to his rituals often resulted in aggressive behaviors. These behaviors interfered with his ability to function. The intervention program designed to reduce Oscar's stereotypic behavior and maximize his gross motor skills included vigorous seasonal physical activities (swimming, skiing, basketball). Oscar was also placed in music therapy activities twice a week to increase his attention, awareness, and concentration and to decrease random and purposeless self-stimulating behavior. The steps to prevent Oscar's physical aggression include developing a daily tangible, written schedule incorporating his choices and interests. This schedule is read with Oscar at different times throughout the day to ensure that Oscar is prepared and that communication is consistent. Oscar is also offered frequent breaks, especially in a busy or crowded environment. When Oscar shows signs of being tense and frustrated, staff encourage him to engage in some form of physical activity. At times, this consists of walking up and down the driveway until he becomes calm. Oscar uses a boxing bag or a pillow to punch. At times, he'll also engage in vigorous weaving and bread kneading and use the cardio equipment available to him as a part of his physical activity plan.

In addition to fostering independence, intervention goals for Oscar include improved communication. Enabling Oscar to communicate his needs and emotions allows him to let staff know his preferences in activities.

Oscar's quality of life was greatly improved by moving to Bittersweet Farms. Living at home kept Oscar from forming relationships outside of his family. Oscar now participates in recreational activities and travel, and is involved with the community. Oscar is now independent in completing many self-care activities. He is currently learning additional self-help skills such as doing his laundry and making nutritious lunches.

Oscar is popular with the staff and enjoys their positive attention. He's developing a sense of humor and is included in social activities. Staff are aware of what triggers Oscar's stress and work to provide an environment that is relaxing and calm. They continue to provide choices, promote independence, and offer purposeful activities.

The active and aerobic nature of the farmstead model has been very important for Oscar. Opportunities for physical activity provide him with an outlet to express his emotions and help him remain calm. All of Oscar's behavioral plans include engaging him in physical activity. Oscar enjoys downhill and cross-country skiing, mountain climbing, swimming, and playing basketball and shuffleboard. He also thrives on the structure, consistency, and partnership components of the Bittersweet model. Each staff member working with Oscar understands how to avoid or minimize situations that serve as triggers for him. The communication and friendships that staff develop with Oscar allow him to trust them and be motivated to complete tasks and participate in new activities. Such outcomes allow Oscar to experience a greater sense of self-determination.

Social Inclusion

Unfriendly vibes often make it difficult for people with autism to feel comfortable participating in their local communities and social gatherings. One study reported that over 80% of adults with autism felt strongly or very strongly that one of the greatest challenges they faced in life resulted directly from other people's lack of acceptance and understanding of their differences (Beardon & Edmonds, 2007). Sensory issues might also get in the way of social inclusion, as many social environments include physical features or situations which may serve as triggers for people with ASD. For some, large spaces and lots of people create situations where they are unable to function. Loud noises and bright lights—often present in social situations—may also serve as triggers.

Due to the lack of social inclusion, many adults with ASD experience loneliness. They tend to have few relationships with people who aren't family members and are aware of and hurt by feelings of isolation. For some, this awareness tends to increase with age (Tobin et al., 2014).

The Bittersweet model uses a variety of strategies to foster social inclusion. Some residents are encouraged to become involved with community volunteer activities, such as assisting at animal shelters. Residents also participate in supported community outings to such places as local parks, libraries, restaurants, and shops. Their participation in group recreational activities on the farm and in the larger community is encouraged. Social inclusion and a sense of belonging are also promoted through engagement in meaningful activities that make valuable contributions to farm and community life. Promoting a sense of belonging is clearly reflected in the way staff and participants work together with mutual assistance and cooperation.

SOCIAL INCLUSION: PAUL'S STORY

Paul participated in Bittersweet's day program for a number of years before he moved to Bittersweet Farms. His parents were interested in residential placement because Paul's periodic rages were becoming more frequent and intense. As a child, Paul attended special education classes at school. In high school, his multi-handicapped classroom was housed at Bittersweet Farms. Paul's handicaps included autism and a moderate intellectual disability. He exhibited limited communication, self-stimulatory behavior, occasional self-abusive behavior, and ritualistic interests and behaviors. While his receptive language skills allow Paul to understand much of what is said, his expressive language consists primarily of echolalia utterances of two to three words. Paul had problems with aggression when he came to Bittersweet, as well as crying for hours at a time. He still continues to cry for long periods of time when there are changes to his schedule.

The intervention program for Paul while he was still in the day program included participation in community outings to such places as the library, grocery store, and fast-food establishments. Specific goals for Paul included increasing his time on task and completing simple tasks (such as making a salad) using picture cards and prompts from staff. Expressive language goals focused on using words to label his feelings and to talk in longer sentences. Conversations were used to help Paul develop an awareness of others.

When Paul was an adolescent, his involvement in the community was restricted. His behavior was unpredictable, and he would run and refuse to leave restaurants, stores, etc. His parents were limited to taking him to parks and drive-through restaurants. Now, Paul participates in small- and large-group activities and attends community activities. Paul now initiates and responds to conversations. He's able to express his needs and interests clearly. Paul can go shopping, be relaxed, and exercise self-control. When Paul came to Bittersweet, he could not interact with others well. Now he is liked by everyone and has fun with staff. He loves spelling for people and singing.

Working in partnership with staff has allowed Paul to develop relationships which give him a sense of community, belonging, and an awareness of others.

Rights

The United Nations Convention on the Rights of Persons with Disabilities was adopted in 2006 and ratified in 2007. More than 100 countries, including the United States, signed up to this convention. While all of the rights outlined in this convention should be available to people on the autism spectrum, four have been identified as generally not available to adults with ASD: (1) "respect for dignity, autonomy, and independence of people with disabilities; (2) non-discrimination; (3) full and effective participation in society; and (4) respect for differences and acceptance of persons with disabilities as part of human diversity" (Robertson, 2010). Each of these rights are recognized as priorities in the Bittersweet model. Robby's story highlights the ways in which the Bittersweet model shows respect for the dignity of individuals with ASD and is effective in promoting their participation in society.

RIGHTS: ROBBY'S STORY

Robby attended special education classes and lived at home before moving to Bittersweet Farms. During high school, he attended a local multi-handicapped classroom which spent two days a week at Bittersweet in the horticultural program. The fact that Robby's mother was the nurse at Bittersweet helped him adjust well to the program, as he could see his mother every day. His mother reported that Robby had some natural musical ability and could read single words. His expressive language, however, was sparse. He also showed an extreme lack of initiative.

When he first moved to Bittersweet, Robby's immediate need was in the area of communication. He did not initiate speech. When upset, he'd make a loud throat-clearing noise. Periods of agitation were generally precipitated by outbursts of temper by other residents. His own temper tantrums usually resulted from staff's attempt to redirect his behavior.

Robby's extreme lack of initiative continued to be a problem for many years after moving to Bittersweet. He needed constant monitoring of important health issues, such as proper eating, drinking, and sleeping. He needed prompting for almost every self-help activity including going to the bathroom. In order to decrease Robby's dependence on verbal prompting and to decrease his self-stimulating and perseverative behaviors, Robby was scheduled to participate in vigorous activities three times a week. These activities changed with the seasons.

Improved language is an ongoing goal of Robby's intervention plan. Robby is reminded to look at people before speaking or interacting with them. He is encouraged to initiate conversation, and situations are set up to promote that. For instance, Robby is sent on errands to take things to certain people on the farm and is then entrusted with a message to deliver on his return.

Robby's musical ability is encouraged through participation in the bell choir. He's also had piano and drum lessons taught by staff. Robby enjoys singing, playing games, doing jigsaw puzzles, going to church, and making crafts. Robby now works well with the staff and is included in cookouts with the friends with whom he works. While Robby tends to be withdrawn, working on art and woodworking projects gives him opportunities to interact with residents and staff and to enjoy their positive responses.

The partnership aspect of Bittersweet has been critical for Robby. Partnering with staff in reciprocal activities has helped Robby become aware of others and encouraged his attempts to communicate. Robby is encouraged to play interactive games and to read and write with staff.

References

Beardon, L., & Edmonds, G. (2007). *The ASPECT consultancy report: A national report on the needs of adults with Asperger syndrome.* Sheffield: Sheffield Hallam University, The Autism Centre.

Bishop-Fitzpatrick, L., Hong, J., Smith, L. E., Makuch, R. A., Greenberg, J. S., & Mailick, M. R. (2016). Characterizing objective quality of life and normative outcomes in adults with autism spectrum disorder: An exploratory latent class analysis. *Journal of Autism and Developmental Disorders, 46*(8), 2707–2719.

Chawla, L. (2015). Benefits of nature contact for children. *Journal of Planning Literature, 30*(4), 433–452.

Gillot, A., & Standen, P. J. (2007). Levels of anxiety and sources of stress in adults with autism. *Journal of Intellectual Disabilities, 11*(4), 359–370.

Masataka, N. (2017). Implications of the idea of neurodiversity for understanding the origins of developmental disorders. *Physics of Life Reviews, 20*, 85–108.

Nussbaum, M. C. (2011). Human capabilities and animal lives: Conflict, wonder, law: A symposium. *Journal of Human Development, 18*(3), 317–321.

Robertson, S. M. (2010). Neurodiversity, quality of life, and autistic adults: Shifting research and professional focuses onto real-life challenges. *Disability Studies Quarterly, 30*(1), 27.

Schalock, R. L. (2004). The concept of quality of life: What we know and do not know. *Journal of Intellectual Disability Research, 48*(3), 203–216.

Strnadova, I., & Evans, D. (2012). Subjective quality of life of women with intellectual disabilities: The role of perceived control over their own life in self-determined behaviour. *Journal of Applied Research in Intellectual Disabilities, 25*(1), 71–79.

Tobin, M. C., Drager, K. D., & Richardson, L. F. (2014). A systematic review of social participation for adults with autism spectrum disorders: Support, social functioning, and quality of life. *Research in Autism Spectrum Disorders, 8*(3), 214–229.

White, K., Flanagan, T. D., & Nadig, A. (2018). Examining the relationship between self-determination and quality of life in young adults with autism spectrum disorder. *Journal of Developmental and Physical Disabilities, 30*(6), 735–754.

8 Evaluation of the Bittersweet Model

Quantitative Results for the Bittersweet Farms Program Evaluation

Prepared for Dr Jeanne Dennler by Nancy Buderer Consulting, LLC.

An evaluation of the Bittersweet Farms model was conducted in 2020 by Dr Nancy Buderer (biostatistician) and Dr Jeanne Dennler (author). The evaluation focused on 20 individuals who entered Bittersweet Farms between 1983 and 2005. They are all long-term residents of Bittersweet, with 34 years the average time in residence on the farm. Information gathered on each individual included reason for admission to Bittersweet, background information and history, main problem requiring intervention, and unique approaches and interventions used to address the problems. This chapter presents the results of the quantitative component of the evaluation. The Appendix provides more detailed descriptions of selected residents and the positive changes they made while at Bittersweet, especially in relation to quality-of-life indicators.

Purpose

The purpose of this internal study was to evaluate changes in problematic behaviors and quality-of-life domains among long-term residents of Bittersweet Farms in order to identify areas where the Bittersweet model is successful and areas for possible improvement.

Methods

A convenience sample of long-term residents was selected by the senior staff. Included were 20 residents who were placed at Bittersweet between 1983 and 2005, and were currently residing there at the time of data collection (2020) or had recently been discharged (two residents had recently died). Using a standardized data collection form, senior staff retrospectively reviewed each of the resident's records in combination with

DOI: 10.4324/9781003271048-9

their own experience and judgment to evaluate the resident's change in problematic behaviors and quality-of-life domains. Staff were instructed to make their judgments based on the resident's individual level and within the context of his or her life within the Bittersweet community.

Problematic behaviors were subjectively categorized using a four-point scale (none, mild, moderate, severe) upon placement at Bittersweet Farms and again at present or discharge. A resident is classified as having improved if his or her score decreased by one point or more (e.g., from moderate to mild, or from moderate to none). The percentage of residents who improved is calculated among the residents who had the problematic behavior at any level (mild, moderate, or severe) at placement.

The improvement in problem severity for each of the quality-of-life domains (Schalock, 2004; 2007) was subjectively categorized using a four-point scale (no improvement, some improvement, substantial improvement, no longer a problem) comparing the present or discharge status to that of the resident upon placement at Bittersweet Farms. A resident is classified as having improved if he or she had made substantial improvement or the quality-of-life domain was no longer a problem. Included were subjects for whom the domain was a problem at placement.

The Vineland-3 tool (Sparrow et al., 2016) was used to assess the residents' current levels of communication, daily living, socialization, and adaptive behavior.

Results

The records of 20 residents who were placed at Bittersweet between 1983 and 2005 were retrospectively evaluated. Their median age at placement at Bittersweet was 21 years. These were long-term residents with a median of 34 years living at Bittersweet. The majority were Caucasian (16) males (17). All residents were autistic with some level of intellectual disability (eight mild, seven moderate, five severe). The common reasons for placement at Bittersweet included: parent(s) unable to care for/cope with at home (15); resident required a great deal of support and structure (1); or parent(s) unable to provide for programming, stimulation, meaningful activity at home (4).

Over half of the residents arrived at the farm with severe anxiety, limited expressive language, obsessive compulsive disorders (OCD), aggression, or withdrawal (Table 8.1). An improvement from placement to present (about 34 years) was noted for every diagnoses. For example, 89% of those who experienced aggression had improved; 85% with anxiety improved; and 84% with OCD improved. Twelve residents arrived at the farm with moderate to severe self-injurious behavior and improvement was seen in nine or 75% of those residents. Lower rates

Table 8.1 Changes in Problematic Behaviors from Placement to Present (or Discharge)

Diagnosis	Level of severity upon placement at Bittersweet				No. residents with this condition at placement	Improvement from placement to present (or discharge) among residents who had this condition upon placement
	None	Mild	Moderate	Severe		Improved by one or more levels
Anxiety	0	1 (5)	7 (35)	12 (60)	20	17 (85)
Short attention span	0 (0)	6 (30)	5 (25)	9 (45)	20	15 (75)
Obsessive/compulsive	1 (5)	2 (10)	4 (20)	13 (65)	19	16 (84)
Withdrawal	1 (5)	3 (15)	6 (30)	10 (50)	19	15 (79)
Aggression	2 (10)	3 (15)	6 (30)	9 (45)	18	16 (89)
Limited expressive language	4 (20)	1 (5)	4 (20)	11 (55)	16	7 (44)
Depressed mood	4 (20)	4 (20)	9 (45)	3 (15)	16	10 (63)
Psychotic symptoms	7 (35)	5 (25)	5 (25)	3 (15)	13	9 (69)
Self-injurious behavior	8 (40)	0 (0)	6 (30)	6 (30)	12	9 (75)
Sleep problems	9 (45)	3 (15)	5 (25)	3 (15)	11	8 (73)
Eating disorders	12 (60)	4 20)	0 (0)	4 (20)	8	4 (50)

Note: Data are presented as *n* (%).

Table 8.2 Improvement in Quality-of-Life Domains from Placement to Present (or Discharge) among Residents for Whom the Domain was a Problem at Placement

	Improvement in problem severity from placement to present (or discharge)			
	No improvement	*Some improvement*	*Substantial improvement*	*No longer a problem*
Emotional well-being				
Contentment	0 (0)	1 (5)	11 (55)	8 (40)
Self-concept	0 (0)	3 (15)	9 (45)	8 (40)
Lack of stress	0 (0)	3 (15)	9 (45)	8 (40)
Interpersonal relations				
Interactions, communications	0 (0)	1 (5)	7 (35)	12 (60)
Relationships	0 (0)	1 (5)	3 (16)	15 (79)
Supports	0 (0)	0 (0)	1 (6)	17 (94)
Material well-being				
Financial status	0 (0)	0 (0)	0 (0)	19 (100)
Employment, meaningful vocational activity	0 (0)	0 (0)	1 (5)	19 (95)
Personal development				
Education, skill development	0 (0)	5 (25)	7 (35)	8 (40)
Personal competence	0 (0)	7 (35)	6 (30)	7 (35)
Performance	0 (0)	4 (20)	7 (35)	9 (45)
Physical well-being				
Health	2 (13)	3 (19)	5 (31)	6 (38)
Activities of daily living	0 (0)	5 (25)	9 (45)	6 (30)
Leisure	0 (0)	0 (0)	5 (31)	11 (69)

(*Continued*)

Table 8.2 Continued

	Improvement in problem severity from placement to present (or discharge)			
	No improvement	*Some improvement*	*Substantial improvement*	*No longer a problem*
Self-determination				
Autonomy or personal control	0 (0)	10 (50)	3 (15)	7 (35)
Goals and personal values	0 (0)	7 (35)	3 (15)	10 (50)
Choices	0 (0)	0 (0)	1 (5)	19 (95)
Social inclusion				
Community integration, participation	0 (0)	2 (10)	0 (0)	18 (90)
Community roles	0 (0)	2 (10)	0 (0)	18 (90)
Social supports	0 (0)	0 (0)	0 (0)	19 (100)
Rights				
Human	0 (0)	0 (0)	0 (0)	20 (100)
Legal	0 (0)	0 (0)	0 (0)	19 (100)

Table 8.3 Vineland-3 Results

	Median (IQR)
Test age	55 (53, 59)
Communication standard score	45 (29, 60)
Daily living skills standard score	42 (30, 63)
Socialization standard score	39 (31, 47)
Sum of domain standard scores	130 (93, 165)
Adaptive behavior composite score	48 (35, 58)
Internalizing raw score (section A)	8 (6, 12)
Externalizing raw score (section B)	4 (3, 7)

Note: IQR is the interquartile range (25th percentile, 75th percentile). Summary statistics are rounded to the nearest whole number. n = 20 subjects.

of improvement were seen with respect to eating disorders (50%) and expressive language (44%) (Table 8.1).

Twenty-two aspects of quality of life were evaluated at the present time in comparison to placement. Of the residents, over 90% showed substantial improvement or the domain was no longer a problem for the following areas: contentment, interactions/communications, relationships, supports, financial status, meaningful vocation, leisure, choices, community integration, community roles, social supports, human rights, and legal rights (Table 8.2). Autonomy or personal control remained a problem for half of the residents.

Using the Vineland-3, the median scores combining all residents showed that as a group, they were more than three standard deviations below the norm (score of 100) with respect to communication, daily living skills, socialization, and adaptive behavior composite score (Table 8.3) (Sparrow et al., 2016).

Discussion

One of the most striking themes to emerge from the data and a review of the clinical records is the diversity of the residents. The residents were similar in that they all had autism, intellectual deficits of varying degrees, and low adaptive behavior scores. But their backgrounds represented a very diverse population, racially and socioeconomically. Some residents came from well-educated, two-parent homes and others from institutions and foster care. Some residents were able to be educated in their local school systems, but others needed hospitalization or institutional placements. Sixteen of the residents came with limited expressive language, of which some were non-verbal. One resident was deaf. The residents were all complex with medical and psychiatric comorbid conditions; some more severe than others. Yet, all 20 residents in the evaluation made significant improvements in their quality of life. This type of transformation suggests that the farmstead model of treatment is effective across differing levels of intellectual, behavioral, communicative, and diagnostic areas.

The change in problematic behaviors from placement to discharge (or death) is presented in Table 8.1. Improvement was noted in every diagnosis. One of the most significant changes was in aggression. Aggression was stated as the most frequent problem area at admission for 18 of the 20 residents. Aggressive behaviors interfered with the resident's ability to participate in group activities and be productive. Of these 18 residents, 16 made improvements by one level or more. The vast majority of people with ASD have sensory processing deficits which are highly correlated with aggression (van den Boogert et al., 2021). Self-injurious behavior is also highly correlated with abnormal sensory processing in children with autism spectrum disorder as well as a need for sameness. The researchers recommended that treatment should focus on these factors (van den Boogert et al., 2021). Twelve residents in this study, when admitted to Bittersweet, demonstrated moderate to severe problems in self-injurious behaviors. Nine of the 12 residents made some level of progress (Table 8.1).

Data on sensory processing disorders were not included in the list of diagnoses or problematic behaviors (Table 8.1) since a sensory processing disorder is not a medical diagnosis and has only been part of the diagnostic criteria for ASD since its inclusion in the *Diagnostic and Statistical Manual of Mental Disorders* (DSM-5) in 2013. In a thorough review of clinical records, there was little mention of sensory processing difficulties when the residents were admitted. Before the late 1990s, occupational therapy assessments and sensory processing recommendations were not included in the clinical records of residents.

The emphasis of the Bittersweet program on heavy farm work and hiking in the woods addresses many of the sensory input needs of the residents. Specific sensory recommendations include long hikes in woods carrying heavy backpacks (filled with food and thermos), chopping wood and collecting sticks for wood-burning stoves, and using wheelbarrows rather than pull carts to receive the maximum proprioceptive input. Physical exercise is associated with a reduction in anxiety (Svensson et al., 2021). Seventeen of the 20 residents included in the evaluation had a reduction in their anxiety. The Bittersweet model of exercise and work associated with sensory input may be related to the improvement in the residents' aggression and anxiety. Further research on the effectiveness of sensory input interventions for reducing aggressive and self-injurious behavior in this population is warranted.

Table 8.2 delineates the changes in eight quality-of-life domains based on the results of a standardized collection form. The eight domains are discussed as follows:

The domain of emotional well-being includes items of contentment, self-concept, and lack of stress. In the area of contentment, all 20 residents made gains with 19 making significant gains. When we look back at Maslow's hierarchy in Chapter 2, we see that contentment falls under self-actualization. This implies that residents' most basic needs for survival have been met by being at the farm. The residents are provided with the safety, security, structure, and routine they need to be calm and productive. The residents become part of a community and feel a sense of belonging and appreciation. Self-concept is a result of mastering skills and feeling a sense of accomplishment. Bittersweet provides purposeful work at different levels so all residents can participate and be successful.

The domain of interpersonal relations includes the items of interactions/communications, relationships, and supports. A key component of the Bittersweet program is the development of relationships between the staff and the residents through the process of partnership. Partnership involves staff working with a resident on a task, not supervising them. In a partnership activity, a relationship develops with reciprocal communication and interactions. Staff provide the support during all tasks and teach vocabulary, language concepts, and social skills. All residents who had problems in this area made significant improvement or no longer had problems with interpersonal relations. The apprenticeship model and partnership (Chapter 4) appear to be critical in improving quality-of-life changes in this area.

The domain of social inclusion is another area where all 20 residents made substantial improvement or no longer had problems in this area. The Bittersweet model promotes interdependence between the staff and residents. Work and leisure activities encourage residents to be involved together in completing tasks which are planned to include a wide range of skills. Social activities at the farm include everyone, and each resident is included in community outings according to his or her level of comfort in that environment. The rural town near the farmstead includes residents in church activities and community events. The emphasis on social inclusion in daily planning gives residents a sense of belonging to a community. On the Maslow hierarchy, becoming part of a community is a critical step toward contentment and self-actualization.

In the domains of material well-being and physical well-being, residents are taken care of by the organization. Bittersweet is a private non-profit and community-supported facility which receives grants and donations. All residents are on some type of social security and that money goes farther at Bittersweet which has a lower operating cost than if they were paying rent in an apartment in town. They all have Medicaid and some have Medicare enabling them to have good health care. In addition, all residents have purposeful employment at their interest and ability level. They are all paid for their work and can save it to go on activities and trips. Those residents who choose to work less still have their special needs and interests met.

Personal development, physical well-being, and self-determination have more varied results. All residents have made progress in having choices because those are provided by the structure of the program. Progress in the areas of autonomy, personal control and daily living skills all require individual competencies. As noted in Table 8.2, autonomy and personal control remained a problem for half the population. Residents vary greatly in their level of intellectual deficits, expressive language, and the degree of sensory processing deficits. One of the core characteristics of autism is restricted or repetitive patterns of thought and behavior, especially in individuals with severe autism. All of these characteristics can interfere with the development of autonomy, personal control and development of independent daily living skills. Individuals with more severe deficits need more support from direct service staff.

The quantitative evaluation of the Bittersweet model has several limitations that should be considered when interpreting the results. This was not a research study, and the results may not be generalizable to other programs. A convenience sample of residents were included which may pose a selection bias. Data were retrospectively abstracted from years of records that were kept for purposes other than this evaluation, and the scoring system was developed specifically for this evaluation without external validity testing. Data abstractors were also Bittersweet staff and their assessments of how residents improved may have been biased.

Recommendations

The Bittersweet model has been successful in improving the quality of life of residents and has been transformative in their lives. But as residents age, the Board of Directors need to plan for the future. Decisions on hospice care and physical and medical conditions related to aging need to be addressed. When residents have been transferred to other facilities, they no longer have the structure and support or trained care givers and their behavior regresses.

As noted above, recent research on sensory processing disorders indicate that the work activities and hiking in the original model of Bittersweet are critical in helping adults with autism reduce their aggression and self-injurious behavior. This is the core of the Bittersweet model which must be preserved and understood by the direct care staff. Emphasis should be put on documenting sensory processing deficits with individual sensory profiles to help direct care staff better understand the residents they partner with and help them provide the enthusiasm and motivation to engage residents in this therapeutic work. Staff training is key in helping them understand and know that they provide critical interventions which impact quality of life.

Summary

The overall results of this evaluation indicate that the Bittersweet Farms model of intervention for adults on the autism spectrum is effective in promoting multiple dimensions of quality of life for the residents. These results can't identify exactly which elements of the Bittersweet model contribute most to enhancing the residents' quality of life, yet related research, staff observations, and responses from the residents indicate that the farm setting with daily engagement with nature, the structure of the day adapted to individual needs and interests, the variety of sensory-rich activities, and the reciprocal relationship with staff play an important role in the process. While more research is needed to document the benefits of the interventions used in the Bittersweet model, the available evidence is strong enough to justify replication of the Bittersweet approach.

References

Schalock, R. L. (2004). The concept of quality of life: What we know and do not know. *Journal of Intellectual Disability Research*, *48*(3), 203–216.

Schalock, R. L., Gardner, J. S., & Bradley, V. J. (2007). *Quality of life for people with intellectual and other developmental disabilities*. Washington, DC: American Association of Intellectual and Developmental Disabilities.

Sparrow, S. S., Cicchetti, D. V., & Saulnier, C. A. (2016). *Vineland adaptive behavior scales- third edition (Vineland-3)*. London: Pearson.

Svensson, M., Brundin, L., Erhardt, S., Hållmarker, U., James, S., & Deierborg, T. (2021). Physical activity is associated with lower long-term incidence of anxiety in a population-based, large-scale study. *Frontiers in Psychiatry*, *12*, 714014–714014.

van den Boogert, F., Sizoo, B., Spaan, P., Tolstra, S., Bouman, Y. H. A., Hoogendijk, W. J. G., & Roza, S. J. (2021). Sensory processing and aggressive behavior in adults with autism spectrum disorder. *Brain Sciences*, *11*(1), 95.

9 Growth of Bittersweet Over the Years

The Bittersweet farmstead and its treatment model have thrived and expanded locally since it opened in 1983. From 20 residents, the farm in Whitehouse now houses 40 residents in different types of housing arrangements, depending on the residents' funding and their individual needs. In 2007, Bittersweet was awarded a 1.3 million dollar grant for construction of 12 new supported living residential units on the Whitehouse property. Twenty individuals now live in the residential program and 20 in supportive living units. Approximately 30 participants, who live with their families or at other institutions, come for a day program, which began when Bittersweet opened. The participants join with residents in the variety of activities found on the farmstead.

An additional 80-acre farm in Lima, Ohio, was willed to Bittersweet in 2006 and is now called "Betty's Farm." Betty's Farm offers a day program that focuses on life and safety skills, aerobic outdoor activities, gardening, civic education, and volunteering in programs in Lima. Volunteer sites include Habitat for Humanity, local parks, and food banks. Vegetables grown on Betty's Farm are donated to families in need and to soup kitchens. The day program is based on the same therapeutic model as Bittersweet Farms and focuses on a daily structure, partnership, and therapeutic and communicative interactions with staff to facilitate language and communication skills. Approximately 15 participants are part of the Lima day program.

In 2007, Bittersweet began providing a transition program for adolescents ages 12–22 in Pemberville, Ohio. Local school districts approached Bittersweet to provide educational services to help students with autism spectrum disorder (ASD) transition to adulthood. A curriculum was developed to meet the unique needs of each student, and an intervention specialist works with the home school, student, and family to foster skills which are academic, with a focus on developing life skills. On completion of the transition program, students receive their high school diploma

DOI: 10.4324/9781003271048-10

from their home district. Bittersweet also offers an extended school year for these students for six weeks during the summer. This program offers camp activities, along with individualized academic enrichment activities.

Bittersweet has developed additional outreach programs for young adults. A social recreational program is held weekly for young adults in the community who can come and socialize while participating in different activities at Bittersweet, such as cooking or going on outings. Typically, ten participants are involved. This program provides additional activities for students who are mainstreamed in their home schools but who need more opportunities to be socially interactive and to develop friendships.

Bittersweet also has several market and mobile ventures. For several years, Bittersweet participants sold vegetables at a local farmer's market. Currently, they grow vegetables and sell them through a community-supported agriculture (CSA) program. They also have a new storefront market on the farm to display and sell produce and goods grown and made by participants. This arrangement provides a forum for participants to work on skills related to stocking, pricing, marketing/selling,

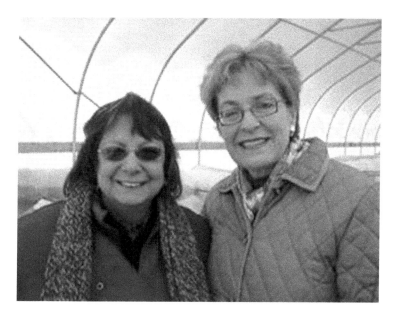

Figure 9.1 Vicki Obee and Congresswoman Marcy Kaptur celebrate the first harvest in the new hoop house at Bittersweet Farms which was used in winter 2007.

and customer interaction and service, as well as inventory management. A "mobile venture" is also in the planning stage for Bittersweet participants. This venture includes the purchase of a mobile trailer unit (somewhat similar to a "food truck") which will be a market on wheels. This unit will take participants' artwork to sell on the road and allow participants to be a part of such community events as art fairs and festivals. Artwork is also sold through Bittersweet's online store, with the proceeds then used to purchase more art supplies. One of the resident artists was commissioned to paint pictures of a purchaser's pets.

The hoop house was built in collaboration with the Center for Innovative Food Technology. This facility allowed the farm to expand its food production and develop a community-supported agriculture (CSA) program, which is now thriving. The program allows participants to be involved with the community. In 2021, the CSA was sold out of shares for spring, summer, and fall. Congresswoman Kaptur has been helpful in supporting Bittersweet in several aspects of its expansion (Figure 9.1).

As Bittersweet participants are aging and "retiring" from work, a new group called Lifestyles has been developed to provide adaptive activities including crafts, community trips, and some physical activity. A changing population requires creative thinking! Regardless of the changes, the components of the model stay the same: structure, partnership, purpose, and activity.

Bittersweet has become known around the world for its innovative farmstead model. People from England, Ireland, Belgium, Japan, Australia, Taiwan, Hungary, Canada, and Russia have come to visit Bittersweet. Many of these visitors have taken part in a week-long class offered at Bittersweet on the components of the model. A team from Taiwan spent ten days at the farm. On returning home, they started the Autism Society of Taiwan and replicated the Bittersweet farmstead model. Vicki Obee, the director of Bittersweet at that time, had the pleasure of witnessing the program in Taiwan when she was invited to be the keynote speaker at the first gathering of the Autism Society of Taiwan.

In the United States, interest in housing, services, and programs for adults with ASD grew rapidly in the late 2000s as more children "aged out" of school programs, and minimal services were available for adults. Bittersweet Farms was the earliest residential farm for adults with autism and has served as a model for other facilities around the world.

Dustin Watkins, the current executive director of Bittersweet Inc., indicated that planning for the aging population is now the primary focus of the organization. His plans include expanding the clinical services at Bittersweet and including specialists who can evaluate the needs of the aging residents, especially when they develop medical or aging problems. Currently, there are two nurses on staff, but they cannot provide 24-hour coverage. These services will need to be expanded if Bittersweet wants to provide hospice and other medical care. The original plan was to have residents spend their whole life at Bittersweet and maintain their community and their quality of life until the end.

Bittersweet has been a leader in providing exceptional programming for youth and adults with autism since the early 1980s. While exceptional programming might be defined in a number of ways, perhaps the strongest indicator of its success can be found in the residents themselves. Some of the residents from the 1980s still live and thrive at Bittersweet Farms. Their ongoing participation in the Bittersweet community attests to the "goodness of fit" between their unique needs and what the Bittersweet model has to offer.

For the residents, Bittersweet is more than a model or a program. It's also more than a farm in a rural setting. Bittersweet, for the residents, is a home and a community, a place where they can be themselves, where their strengths and interests are recognized, and a place where they belong. Bittersweet is aptly named. In the plant world, bittersweet is a vine, and vines need supports to grow. Given the necessary support, a bittersweet vine can grow up to more than 20-feet in height. It can also flower and bear fruit. For adults with autism, the Bittersweet Farm community provides the support they need in order to enjoy a quality of life in sync with their unique way of being in the world.

Epilogue
Why Bittersweet?

Since 1983, Bittersweet Farms, sitting on 80 acres of farmland and forest, has been a safe haven for adults with autism who have severe outward behaviors and who did not fit into traditional residential settings. A recent program evaluation profiled 20 residents who have been living at Bittersweet for over 30 years. A quality-of-life scale developed for this population was used to measure improvements over time. The results—as presented in this book about Bittersweet Farms—are overwhelmingly positive.

Parents on the board of directors for Bittersweet Farms requested that this book be written to preserve in writing the therapeutic model which enabled their children to thrive and to live in a humane setting focused on their children's talents and needs. Of the 20 residents profiled, 18 entered the farmstead with severe aggressive and self-injurious behaviors. Their parents or their residential providers were unable to provide structure or manage their extreme outward behaviors which included hitting, throwing objects, attempting to harm others, throwing themselves on the ground, and biting themselves and others. All 20 residents had additional diagnoses including intellectual deficits and severe sensory processing deficits. Many residents had additional psychiatric diagnoses, such as obsessive-compulsive disorders, eating disorders, withdrawal, and short attention spans. Many had limited expressive language, and all had problems with communication.

The farm provides a setting that addresses the residents' sensory processing disorders—a major contributor to their aggressive behaviors. The hard physical work of the farm provides proprioceptive and vestibular input in such purposeful activities as feeding the animals, chopping wood, and hauling loads of wood to the woodshed and greenhouse which are heated by wood stoves. Hiking daily for 2 or 3 miles and on Saturdays for up to 12 miles provides aerobic exercise, along with sensory input in a calming setting. Carrying something heavy while hiking—such as backpacks filled with thermoses and snacks for breaks—provides additional proprioceptive input. Walking on horse trails with sand and navigating other types of terrain also provide sensory experiences while promoting balance and coordination.

The structure of life on the farm is unique and allows for individual choices not found in traditional therapeutic settings. A wide variety of tasks provide meaningful work for all levels of functioning. One resident can be maintaining the motor of the riding mower used for mowing large areas while another resident can push an old-fashioned mower without the loud noise or smell of gas. In the greenhouses and outdoor landscape, one resident can design the flower beds while others may need help planting seeds and transplanting young vegetables into the outdoor beds. Each resident works at his or her own pace. Some residents with short attention spans need help staying on task while others may need to run outside for a while if overstimulated by the activity or the group. At times, a resident's behavior may regress to the point of needing an evaluation and specific intervention. When this occurs, the work they were doing waits for them; and they can return to it when they are more stable. Community-based work settings are generally not this flexible. A person whose behavior regresses at work usually loses his or her job and work site community. At Bittersweet, where community is a central goal, residents are always supported regardless of their ability to be productive. The staff at Bittersweet are trained in autism and learn how to respond to each resident's individual needs.

Traditional settings may have individuals with different developmental disabilities all in one housing and workplace. The staff in such settings may not have specific training in autism and thus use general interventions that might trigger aggression in a person with autism. Bittersweet works from a partnership model, meaning that staff do not supervise residents but work as partners in all tasks. This process promotes positive relationships which are critical for building a sense of community.

Creating Quality of Life for Adults on the Autism Spectrum: The Story of Bittersweet Farms outlines the many unique features of Bittersweet which have proven successful in helping individuals with autism enjoy a sense of well-being and happiness not possible for them in more traditional settings.

Thousands of families struggle with the challenges of raising autistic children and worry about their future after they age out of school programs. Bittersweet Farms has demonstrated success with a small group of participants and the program has already been copied around the world. Replication requires funding, family commitment, and a desire to provide these amazing individuals with a productive and purposeful life.

A thorough review of the clinical records of the 20 residents in the study suggests that several types of professionals have been important to the success of the Bittersweet treatment model.

A full-time speech therapist at Bittersweet has been critical in increasing residents' communication and social interaction. In the clinical records, there are multiple examples of the speech therapist developing treatment plans and then training the direct care staff to work with residents to increase their vocabulary, understand concepts, develop reciprocal communication patterns, model social greeting, social skills, etc., while working in partnership. With a full-time speech therapist on staff, training was ongoing. The speech therapist was also helpful in developing behavioral interventions when limited language skills contributed to a resident's frustration, often triggering aggressive behaviors. Speech therapists are trained in diverse areas which make them important resources for people with ASD. Speech therapists have the knowledge and skill to address language (understanding and use), social pragmatic language (social language skills we use in our daily interactions with others including non-verbal communication), pre-language, and non-verbal communication, and develop functional communication using alternative and augmentative communication (AAC). These areas have all been essential in working with the adults at Bittersweet.

In adults with autism, sensory abnormalities were present in 94% of the population (Crane et al., 2009). With adults with autism spectrum disorders (ASD) who need more structure and support, sensory processing abnormalities are relatively universal and can be very disabling (Gonthier et al., 2016). There is a strong association between sensory processing and aggressive behaviors. These statistics, found in Chapter 5, speak to the need for an occupational therapist on the staff of a farmstead. Occupational therapy assessments of sensory functioning have allowed Bittersweet staff to develop specific programs for individuals to receive the sensory input they need to function calmly in a community.

> In sum, clinical practice may benefit from applying a detailed assessment of sensory processing problems when treating aggressive behavioral problems in adults with ASD. Therapist and patients may use the sensory profile as an alternative treatment target in case of unexplained or treatment-resistant aggressive behaviors.
>
> (van den Boogert et al., 2021)

Occupational therapists are trained in many areas, including developing sensory processing profiles and diagnosing sensory processing disorders.

In addition to working with sensory processing disorders, occupational therapists are trained to work with disabled, ill, or injured patients with special equipment who need therapeutic support for daily activities. They may provide long-term or acute patient care. If a residential facility plans to provide adults with autism with a lifelong community where they can enjoy a greater quality of life, occupational therapists and nursing staff will need to be employed. When residents are sent to other care facilities where staff are not trained to work with people with autism who often have significant behavioral problems, residents usually regress in their behaviors.

A multidisciplinary team of specialists, including psychologist, psychiatrists, behavioral specialists, speech therapists, occupational therapists, and medical staff, need to support the direct care staff in developing individual plans and interventions.

It is my heartfelt desire that this book will be useful to the families and children who wrestle with autism and to the professionals who support them. It has been my pleasure to work with the Bittersweet staff and to get to know the gifted residents who have the opportunity to live in a beautiful natural setting. Bittersweet is a story filled with hope!

Jeanne Dennler, PhD

References

Crane, L., Goddard, L., & Pring, L. (2009). Sensory processing in adults with autism spectrum disorders. *Autism*, *13*(3), 215–228.

Gonthier, C., Longuépée, L., & Bouvard, M. (2016). Sensory processing in low-functioning adults with autism spectrum disorder: Distinct sensory profiles and their relationships with behavioral dysfunction. *Journal of Autism and Developmental Disorders*, *46*(9), 3078–3089.

van den Boogert, F., Sizoo, B., Spaan, P., Tolstra, S., Bouman, Y. H. A., Hoogendijk, W. J. G., & Roza, S. J. (2021). Sensory processing and aggressive behavior in adults with autism spectrum disorder. *Brain Sciences*, *11*(1), 95.

Glossary

Adaptive behavior: Everyday behavior that enables a person to function well in his or her environment.

Affordances: Qualities or properties of an object or environment that define its possible uses.

Aggression: Hostile or violent behavior or attitude that is—or can be—harmful to others.

Augmentative and alternative communication/assistive speech devices (ASD):   Forms of communicating which do not involve speech, such as sign language, pictures, or speech-generating devices (SGD).

Autism spectrum disorder (ASD):   A broad term encompassing the general form of autism as well as several related disabilities sharing many of the same characteristics.

Biophilia: Instinctive bond between human beings and other living organisms and systems; innate affinity for the natural world.

Communication device: Hardware, such as an iPad, that allows a person who has difficulty communicating using his or her voice to use words or symbols for communication. May range in complexity from a simple picture board to complex electronic devices.

Direct support professional: A person who works directly with people with disabilities with the aim of assisting the individual to become integrated into his or her community.

Echolalia: The echoing and repetition of a phrase or word.

Eco-psychosomatics: The study of the close connection between body, mind, and nature.

Eudaimonic well-being: A descriptor for human flourishing or functioning well as an individual.

Executive functioning: A set of cognitive processes that gives an individual cognitive control over his or her behavior, such as attentional control, cognitive inhibition, inhibitory control, working memory, and cognitive flexibility.

Form: Manifestation. The form of a behavior is the way a person behaves.

Function: The reason why something happens. The function of a behavior is what motivates the behavior.

Functional assessment: An evaluation designed to determine the relationship between what occurs in an individual's environment and the occurrence of challenging behaviors.

Generalization: The ability to perform the same activity in a variety of settings.

Hedonic well-being: A descriptor for feeling well or having pleasant feelings.

Hypersensitive: Being overly sensitive to sensory stimulation.

Hyposensitive: Being under-sensitive to sensory stimulation.

Maladaptive behavior: A behavior that interferes with successful functioning in one's environment.

Neurodiverse: A label sometimes used for people displaying or characterized by autistic or other neurologically atypical patterns of thought or behavior; not neurotypical.

Neurotypical/neurologically typical: A label sometimes used for people who are not on the autism spectrum or for people who show no other neurologically atypical patterns of thought or behavior.

Occupational therapy: A profession within the healthcare system designed to help individuals develop, recover, or maintain meaningful activities required for successful functioning in different environments. Occupational therapists also evaluate and treat sensory processing disorders.

Proprioceptive sense: The sense that informs an individual about where his or her parts of the body are and what they are doing.

Quality of life: An individual's perception of his or her position in life as it relates to health, comfort, and happiness; often defined in relation to eight domains: interpersonal relations, social inclusion, personal development, physical well-being, self-determination, material well-being, emotional well-being, and human and legal rights.

Ritualistic behavior: A behavior that follows a set pattern or routine without variation; usually involves behaviors that are not logical.

Self-regulation: The ability to monitor and modulate one's emotions and behaviors.

Self-stimulation: Involves behaviors motivated by the desire or need to get extra sensory input.

Sensory integration: The ability to feel and understand sensory data from the environment and from one's own body; the ability to analyze and respond appropriately to information received through the senses.

Sensory processing disorder: A condition in which an individual has trouble receiving and responding to information that comes in through the senses; the inability to regulate information received through the senses.

Stereotypic behavior: Behavior that is carried out repeatedly which involves movement of one's body or of an object.

Vestibular sense: The sense that provides information about balance, gravity, and movement.

Appendix

The Appendix includes the profiles of individuals who entered Bittersweet Farms between 1983 and 2005. They are all long-term residents of Bittersweet, with 34 years being the average time at Bittersweet. Each profile includes reason for admission to Bittersweet, background information and history about the resident, main problem requiring intervention, and unique approaches and interventions used to address the problems. Also included with each profile is a description of quality of life (QOL) changes experienced by the resident while at Bittersweet and a discussion about how the Bittersweet model was able to help the resident more so than other traditional intervention models could do. A few of the profiles include a brief summary of a recent interview conducted with the resident. The names of the residents have been changed.

The discussion about quality-of-life changes is based on the Bittersweet Farms evaluation conducted by Dr Nancy Buderer and Dr Jeanne Dennler in 2020. Quality of life is sometimes defined and measured in relation to eight domains: interpersonal relations, social inclusion, personal development, physical well-being, self-determination, material well-being, emotional well-being, and human and legal rights. Each of these domains was considered in the evaluation of the Bittersweet model.

Adam

Reason for Admission

Adam's parents were unable to care for him at home after his behavior became oppositional and he began wandering in the neighborhood.

Background Information and History

Adam lived at home with his family until his placement at Bittersweet in 1988 at the age of 18. Adam has autism, an obsessive-compulsive disorder (OCD), and functions in the mild intellectual disability range. His expressive language was limited to simple declarative statements and questioning sentences, yet he was able to comprehend complex language. Adam attended special education classes until he graduated from high school. In ninth grade, he was in a more inclusive program, where he was teased and taunted and once had his coat-burned by other students. Adam's behavior deteriorated and he lost interest in activities and became oppositional. His withdrawal increased, and he became more preoccupied with bizarre ideas and psychotic thinking. His physical behavior included more motor stereotypes, including spending long periods rocking and jerking, indicating a significant problem with his sensory processing. Adam was transferred to a more structured setting at another high school with a classroom for children with autism. Adam had been attending summer programs and high school classes at Bittersweet as part of his special education class. After exposure to the farm program, Adam expressed an interest in living there. When he arrived at Bittersweet, he had limited social skills, awareness of expectations, and when given too much freedom would be socially inappropriate and aggressive. Adam became oppositional when he felt he was being confronted or challenged. In one reported incident, Adam would not move out of the road when directly asked even when there was ongoing traffic.

Main Problem

Adam had problems with outbursts, aggression, and oppositional behavior particularly at times of stress, instruction, or correction. For example, early on at the farm there had been an issue that made Adam angry, and he rode off on a bicycle into the neighborhood. He was found by a staff member who saw his bicycle outside an old schoolhouse. Adam had broken into the building and hid behind the driver's seat of an old grain truck.

Unique Approaches and Interventions

The highly structured environment at the farm helped Adam develop self-control. By 1993, both the frequency and the intensity of Adam's outbursts had significantly decreased. Adam participates in tasks in horticulture, the barn, landscaping, and the workshop—all of which provide him with needed sensory input. Adam has vestibular deficits and needs a great deal of movement, such as rocking. He also demonstrates tactile defensiveness and does not like to wear clothes.

He will often wear just shorts and tank tops in all types of weather. Meeting Adam's sensory needs helps reduce his aggression. The staff provide Adam with options throughout the day, and he can choose activities which interest him the most. Adam does not like to feel forced or challenged into doing something he does not want to do or understand. Partnership has helped Adam be less aggressive because he feels he is understood. Adam had frequent problems with urinary incontinence, occasional fecal incontinence, and also frequently tore his clothes. These behaviors were reinforced by attention from the staff and a behavior program was developed to involve time away from attention. In 1991, Adam showed deficits in judgment, comprehension, and social cause and effect. His urinary and fecal incontinence was less, happening only when he was angry. Adam has to be supervised for pica (eating items other than food) and other harmful actions. He purposefully stepped on a spike in a board and had to be taken to the emergency room. These behaviors impact his ability to be independent. Adam tends to hoard items, usually soaps, disinfectants, cleaners, or cooking spray. He has also hoarded spray paint, rodent killer, ant bait, ammonia, moth balls, nail polish remover, and turpentine. He may hide these items not only in his room but also in other rooms, storage areas, heating/cooling vents, and in the woods. The staff have very strict rules about what he keeps in his room. These are ongoing behaviors that are managed by behavioral plans.

Quality-of-Life Changes

Adam made substantial improvement in all areas of the eight quality-of-life domains, although he made minimal progress in some items within the domains. Adam is concerned about what is fair and equal. He will say "thank you for understanding" and "thank you for seeing things my way." He is focused on his rights and is his own advocate. This is representative of the QOL domain of "rights" in the domain of self-determination. Yet, limits are placed on Adam's independence. For example, once when his parents took him to a mall, his behavior became inappropriate, and the police were called. There were two other incidents with his parents when Adam exhibited inappropriate behavior which could have led to an arrest. However, in response to the structure of the farm model and his relationships with staff, Adam is now able to be appropriate in the community with supervision. Adam requires 24-hour supervision and is never in the community without a staff member. Under the self-determination domain, Adam has improved significantly in that he can be given choices and can set personal goals. Adam made significant gains in the domains of emotional well-being, interpersonal relations, personal development, and social inclusion. Adam is interested in all outings provided by Bittersweet and took art lessons at a local community college. Although he is not interested in participating in sports, Adam is in the Special Olympics pep club and enjoys cheering for other residents. He is very social and involved with the Bittersweet community. He enjoys mixing beverages together, discussing human rights, and shopping. Adam enjoys contemporary and country music and coffee. He has a strong sense of humor and is socially motivated. Despite Adam's continuing behavior problems, he is able to participate in activities, enjoy meaningful relationships, and have choices in social and work activities. In the domain of physical well-being, Adam has made minimal progress in the self-care areas. He also struggles with anorexia. In the leisure area, he no longer has any problems and enjoys many recreational activities.

Discussion

Bittersweet's attention to residents' sensory needs in their work program and hiking in the woods has greatly benefited Adam. Other work settings could not have provided these interventions to the extent available at Bittersweet. Sensory processing deficits are associated with aggression in people with autism. Partnership has been critical for Adam. Adam's relationships with the staff and their willingness to discuss his actions and give him explanations for rules have also reduced Adam's aggression and acting out behavior. Speech therapy goals in communication and pragmatics have been helpful for Adam and attest to the benefit of having a speech therapist on staff who specializes in autism. The staff can tell Adam that the items he hoards may be dangerous for other residents and that is why he cannot have the items in his room or where he is working. He is more compliant when he understands these ramifications. Adam appears to be happy and content and seems to enjoy his life at the farm.

Interviewed on October 28, 2020, Adam said he likes the animals, hiking in the forest preserves, and in a camp nearby. He participates in track and field and baseball in the Special Olympics. He likes to cook and works in the barn and horticulture. He likes art therapy and groundskeeping. When asked if there was anything he would change, Adam said that some policies in the Special Olympics could be changed. He is interested in his rights. He likes pep club at the Special Olympics and is excited that basketball practice is starting up. He can cheer for the team!

Alice

Reason for Admission

Alice was 43 years old when she moved to Bittersweet in 1992. Prior to that, she had lived her entire life with her parents. Her parents wanted Alice to live in a structured environment with more enrichment than they could provide at home.

Background Information and History

Alice is the younger of two children. She was uncommunicative at the age of four and was diagnosed as autistic. She has a mild intellectual disability. Alice attended regular education classes in public and parochial school and received average grades. Her adjustment to school was difficult and she was not accepted into any peer group. At school, she was picked on, and boys played cruel jokes on her. Alice had two placements at the Toledo Mental Health Center in 1974 and 1975–1976. Alice is legally blind, has no vision in her left eye, and is very near-sighted in her right eye. She has a club foot and Type II diabetes. Alice has good receptive and expressive language skills. She is fairly independent with daily living activities, although she does require some supervision for specific tasks.

Main Problem

Alice's behavior can be explosive and aggressive. She has an obsessive-compulsive disorder and obsessively hoards objects. She verbally and physically attacks people and does not comply with scheduled tasks. Alice used to throw herself down, kick, spit, scream, and yell.

Unique Approaches and Interventions

Behavior modification programming helped Alice develop a basic level of adaptation to the farm. At first, Alice exhibited oppositional behavior and resistance to structure and authority. She resisted group activities and peer interaction. She frequently refused to participate in activities both in her day program and in the evenings and at weekends. After four years of living at Bittersweet, the staff developed a plan for Alice's hoarding that she agreed to. Based on the fire code, residents are only allowed a certain number of items in their room. Alice was allowed to collect whatever she wanted, but she was asked to choose the same number of items to remove from her room. She was, however, unable to go to the donation center herself but would allow a staff member to do so. As long as the staff continued trading objects with her, the interactions usually went smoothly. There were times, however, when her attachment to items would lead to explosive behaviors. Because Alice was diabetic, she had a restrictive diet. At times, Alice would take food to her room and become explosive when confronted with this unacceptable behavior.

The behavioral intervention plan for Alice included treating her with respect and dignity. The staff try to establish a positive and ongoing rapport with Alice regarding her work, interests, and her daily life. They recognize the importance of acknowledging and discussing her frustrations, but also realize that Alice needs limits on her behavior, especially in regard to hoarding. If Alice is found digging through the trash, taking things to her room, putting them in her pockets, or going through items belonging to other people, the staff try to empathize with her and negotiate what can be done with the items. Alice can be very verbally abusive if anyone crosses her and, at times, uses shockingly violent language. Interventions for Alice's verbal outbursts include praising her for appropriate interactions.

Alice's behavior plan specifies rewarding her for following the schedule willingly and being polite. It also helps her develop a sense of responsibility.

At one time, Alice's verbal outbursts were frequent; but after her health improved and her diabetes was under control, Alice herself admitted that it was not worth it to be so angry. She used art to express her feelings. When Alice is given age-appropriate choices in activities and given some control, she is better able to manage her behavior. In 1999, after seven years of living at Bittersweet, Alice averaged 5 incidents of aggression per month and 2.8 incidents of verbal abuse. This was a significant improvement on the previous year.

Alice is capable of holding a grudge. Twelve years ago, Alice told one staff member that she would never speak to her again and she hasn't! When she needs to communicate with this staff member, Alice will write a note! Counseling by the staff has helped Alice deal with conflicts with others. Because Alice is so verbal, she can understand how her behaviors impact others. Alice learned that if she changes her behaviors, she is rewarded with friendships. Alice continues to be motivated by relationships with the staff and responds well when a favorite staff member invites her to work with him or her.

In 2007, Alice was given three goals. The first goal was to develop the ability at a moderate level to self-monitor her own behavior and deal with her environment appropriately. Specifically, this meant learning to express her anger or frustration either verbally, written, or in some other acceptable manner. This also meant using emotional tools to deal with conflict appropriately rather than initiate self-injurious behaviors or become aggressive or destructive. The second goal was to develop the ability to maintain her living quarters in an orderly, clean, and uncluttered manner. The third goal was to be able to maintain personal hygiene with only periodic reminders, including self-care routines and wearing clean clothing. Alice met these goals and is now living in a supported housing unit on the Bittersweet grounds and enjoying her independence.

Quality-of-Life Changes

Alice has made significant progress in all eight QOL domains. The staff view Alice as having blossomed at Bittersweet. When she arrived, she was angry, aggressive, and oppositional defiant. Now, she only demonstrates mild problematic behaviors and psychiatric symptoms. In the domains of interpersonal relations and social inclusion, she has made excellent progress. Alice was very demanding and controlling of other residents. She would criticize them and tell them what to do. She has learned how she could help other residents and she feels better about herself. She learned to contribute in ways that made her feel good as well as make others feel good. Alice is social, now interested in other people, and enjoys many friendships.

In the domain of emotional well-being, Alice feels contentment and satisfaction. Her artwork brings her praise, and she feels accomplished and recognized. In the personal development and self-determination domains, Alice is productive and competent and has a great deal of independence to make many choices.

Within the supportive and structured environment of Bittersweet, Alice has an independent and satisfying life.

Discussion

The most critical part of the Bittersweet model for Alice is partnership. She needs proper social supports to engage in positive relationships and to control her hoarding. The staff are trained to learn about each person and his or her needs and to treat each resident with the kind of respect that encourages residents to comply with the scheduled activities. This type of interaction has had a positive impact on Alice. The Bittersweet focus on exercise and outdoor activity has helped Alice control her diabetes. Alice goes on hikes, walks the track, and walks between vocational areas at the farm which are spaced out over several acres. A farmstead setting has allowed Alice to become healthy and maintain that health compared to a more sedentary environment like a workshop.

The Bittersweet model encourages residents to make choices about their activities until they find areas which are meaningful to them. Alice participates in production art projects during specified times which produce salable art. Her art is used for stationary, and her drawings have been shown in exhibitions around the community. Her art gives her purpose and builds her self-esteem. Alice experiences full quality of life at Bittersweet. She is part of a supportive community and has friendships with staff who help her manage conflict with others. This type of quality of life could not be obtained in other traditional facilities.

Interview Notes

During an interview on October 30, 2020, Alice said that she likes Bittersweet, especially her own little apartment where she now lives. When asked what she likes to do here, she says she mostly likes art. She often paints what other people draw. In the 1990s, when she first came to Bittersweet, Alice worked in the gardens and helped with landscaping. But now that she is retired, she mostly enjoys art. When asked if there was anything she would change about Bittersweet, she said no. She likes everything here, especially her apartment. During the interview, Alice greeted people walking by and was interested in what they were doing. She asked a staff member to go into her apartment and bring out some of her art for me. She showed a lot of pride when showing her art.

Ben

Reason for Admission

Ben's parents could not provide the necessary support and structure Ben needed to function at home.

Background Information and History

Ben, a quiet man, currently functioning at the prevocational level, arrived at Bittersweet in 1987 when he was 19 years old. Prior to entering Bittersweet, Ben was often at risk because of his wandering and inattention to traffic and machinery. Without a structured residential placement, Ben could have been injured and/or required police intervention as a result of his wandering into other people's homes.

Upon placement, Ben had moderate challenges because of his limited expressive language, sleep problems, self-injurious behavior, short attention span, and a moderate intellectual disability. His ability to remain on task was sporadic, even with close supervision and structure. In addition, he had severe challenges, such as anxiety, agitation, obsessive-compulsive behaviors, and eating problems, which caused additional safety issues. Sensory processing deficits contributed to his preference for isolation and his proclivity for agitation, which interfered with his ability to interact effectively with his peers.

Main Problem

One of Ben's biggest issues when he arrived at Bittersweet was maintaining his safety. Ben would wander off the grounds and attempt to consume unsafe foods/items. Initially, Ben would leave the property and be found in a neighbor's house eating from his or her refrigerator.

Unique Approaches and Interventions

To maintain Ben's safety, Bittersweet has provided a setting with 24-hour supervision. Currently, a staff member must keep him in sight at all times and follow him if he attempts to run off. A door alarm is used in the evenings so a staff member is alerted if Ben wanders out of the house. When Ben came to Bittersweet, he would run off the property to a house where he would find food to eat. He seemed to be motivated by cookies and pop. His episodes of running off did not appear to be triggered by anxiety or agitation but simply by opportunity. He would wait until the staff were distracted and then run off.

Over the years, various methods have been investigated, including using a motion alarm, researching personal location devices (such as a Wander Guard Alarm), and finally installing a front gate and fence. Finding a way to contain Ben was critical because without success, he would need to be placed in an institution. At one point, Ben was moved from a 15-bed home to an 8-bed home to provide more supervision. He was given one-on-one supervision, which had many positive benefits in addition to keeping him from running off. These benefits included more physical activity and more positive attention from the staff. Ben's communication skills improved, increasing his ability to express his needs. Most importantly, staff members know that they are held accountable for adhering to Ben's supervision requirements. Ben can still occasionally be seen running off from a work setting with a staff member following him, but his wandering behaviors have decreased significantly as a result of the above interventions.

Ben's agitation was addressed by adding activities where he received proprioceptive input, such as carrying buckets of water to the horses, hiking in the woods, and chopping wood and hauling it to the farm's wood burning stoves.

Quality-of-Life Changes

Ben made substantial gains in seven of the eight QOL domains. When Ben arrived at Bittersweet, his anxiety, short attention span, and agitation were limiting his ability to be happy and content with his surroundings. Gains in the domains of emotional well-being and social inclusion allow Ben to participate in community activities. He no longer lashes out at people when frustrated or anxious. While Ben continues to be at a prevocational level of functioning in some areas, gains in the domains of personal development and self-determination allow him to complete tasks with the help of staff. He still needs assistance in self-care tasks, but enjoys making some choices and exercising some level of independence. Ben's anxiety has been substantially reduced and his communication has improved, increasing his social inclusion. Ben is always treated with respect as he partners with staff in accomplishing tasks. Most importantly, partnering keeps Ben safe from wandering off and hurting himself. For leisure, Ben enjoys ice skating, skiing, and Special Olympics soft ball.

Discussion

Bittersweet allows Ben to have structure and scheduled daily activities to keep him involved in meaningful tasks to avoid perseverating on anxiety-provoking concerns and obsessive-compulsive behaviors. Despite his short attention span and obsessive-compulsive behaviors, the farm setting allows Ben to focus on animals and the concrete tasks of feeding and caring for them. Ben does well in other hands-on areas, such as grounds-keeping where he can get sensory input from pushing, pulling, and other gross motor activities. In all areas of work, Ben interacts with the staff as a partner, taking turns, and hearing the staff describe the tasks they share. In the barn, Ben can watch a staff member measure out the food for an animal and then he can carry it over to the animal stall. The partnership component of the Bittersweet model provides Ben with social interaction, language opportunities, and friendships.

The farm setting has provided Ben with varied tasks that are meaningful to his daily life. Ben has also benefitted from the calmness of the natural setting and the acres of land for walking and getting exercise. Ben's behavior plan includes a variety of interventions that a farmstead situation can offer: changing settings and having him choose different activities, taking him for a walk or a hike, and focusing on vigorous physical activities to reduce his anxiety and stereotypic behavior.

At one point, Ben became agitated when a decorative peace pole was moved on the grounds during the construction of new housing. Ben was upset about the pole being in the wrong place. Different interventions to help Ben deal with the change were not successful. Eventually, the pole was removed to calm him down. This response reflects the philosophy at Bittersweet—the environment can be changed to accommodate the residents. At an institution, this type of flexibility would be limited and would trigger ongoing anxiety and agitation for someone like Ben.

Don

Reason for Admission

Don's mother died in the 1980s and his father was unable to care for him. Subsequently, he went to live with his sister and her family. However, he became aggressive and had self-injurious behaviors, and it was no longer safe for him to be with his sister's family. This resulted in his placement in a group home, where his aggressive and self-injurious behaviors continued. His next placement was in a center for the developmentally disabled. While at this facility, Don participated in the day program at Bittersweet Farms for several years. In 2005, Don, at age 34, was admitted to the Bittersweet residential program.

Background Information and History

Don has good receptive language skills, but cannot speak. He can vocalize and use sign language. When Don entered Bittersweet he had severe anxiety, aggression, and self-injurious behaviors. Don has a moderate intellectual disability. He is fairly independent with most daily living skills although he is slow in completing these tasks. Don had many sensory processing deficits which needed to be addressed. He has a very good memory and will remember sequences.

Major Problem

Don's major problems were severe aggression and self-injurious behaviors. He would throw himself on the ground, bite chunks out of his hand, and bang his head. When Don first came to Bittersweet, he would exhibit these behavior approximately four times a week. Don would throw himself down so hard that eventually he needed back surgery.

Unique Approaches and Interventions

Don's sensory processing needs are addressed through daily hiking and jobs on the farm. His jobs include stacking wood, mulching, hauling brush, and mowing with a push mower which provides proprioceptive input. Regular exercise is part of Don's daily schedule and an important part of his intervention plan. Even when the weather is cold or rainy, he goes to the track for an extended walk. Don also uses the indoor bike. If Don shows signs of self-injurious behavior, he is encouraged to walk the track three or four times that day. Going outside to calm down is part of his behavior plan. Don's agitation and self-injurious behavior are often triggered by anxiety about his schedule. He has responded well to the structure at the farm and needs to know what will be happening next. When Don is upset, his assigned staff implement the following:

1. Staff will communicate with Don and offer redirection or intervention. At times, this also means modifying his environment to make it less overstimulating. His sensory needs must always be considered.
2. Staff will remain calm and relaxed.
3. Staff will ask Don how he can be helped by giving him choices. "Would you rather we… or…?"
4. Staff will recognize and acknowledge Don's answer, and be sincere and honest with him about what is going on.
5. If Don wants something that is not immediately available, staff will *not* ask him to wait. The staff will offer choices of activities he can complete in the area and tell Don when the desired activity will be occurring, referring to his schedule as needed.

The staff try to talk to Don in short sentences and use humor and smiles. They complement his successful attempts to communicate to others. Don does not like to be talked "at" and the staff share conversations with him and treat him intelligently and honestly as a peer. Preventively, staff encourage Don to be in environments which limit, or are free from, loud noises, uncomfortable lighting, and crowds. The staff will offer Don to take breaks in other areas until the noise or crowds subside. They also offer Don headphones to wear in loud environments or use of a sound machine or fan, especially during the overnight hours.

Quality-of-Life Changes

Don has made substantial gains in all eight QOL domains. Being part of the calm and structured Bittersweet environment has reduced Don's aggression and self-injurious behaviors significantly. He is still mildly anxious, but this is also significantly reduced. As a result of these improvements in his mental health and emotional well-being, Don can now safely participate—with the appropriate social supports—in more social settings. Don has made gains in the domains of emotional well-being and interpersonal relations. Don no longer has problems in the domain of social inclusion. He enjoys going out into the community. He loves shopping and buying sparkling water. He loves parades! Don is not involved in sports, but he enjoys being part of the pep club at the Special Olympics. On Wednesdays, he goes to a church community lunch. Don cleans the church on Mondays as his donation to the church. Bittersweet donates extra vegetables to the church and sometimes Don will get to eat what he has helped to grow. This gives Don satisfaction and purpose. He has made gains in the domain of personal development in his sense of achievement and productivity. Don likes to look through catalogs, and collect pamphlets and pictures from places he has visited. He enjoys baking. Don enjoys being outside and this is very calming for him. He enjoys Pizza Hut, Frisch's Big Boy, and going to his sister's house. He has also been involved with sporting events, camping, and water parks. He now has many choices in his life and has made gains in the domain of self-determination.

Discussion

Don has responded well to the structure of the farm, and he likes to know what is going on and what will happen next. Don is at a prevocational level and has a very short attention span. He is not focused on work, but he enjoys watching people work! The Bittersweet model allows for different levels of skills and participation. The farmstead allows opportunities for Don to engage in proprioceptive and vestibular activities to address his sensory needs. Activities are chosen which include bending, stretching, swinging, rocking, hiking in the woods, and walking on the track. Being in a seated position for long periods of time—as Don would be in a workshop setting—would be counterproductive. The variety of activities at the farm allows Don to choose his preference of work sites. He enjoys arts and crafts and baking. Don has worked in the barn and in other nature-based areas. His vocational tasks include animal care, crop production, horticulture, recreational activities, and craft production.

Partnership has helped Don increase his expressive communication. He has learned signs easily. His increased ability to communicate has allowed him to be more interactive and to get his needs met. Don has profited from the presence of a speech therapist on the staff. He now has staff whom he trusts and has learned to develop friendships. The focus on outdoor activities and aerobic exercise has been a critical part of Don's treatment. Exercise and being in an outdoor setting help him remain calm and less aggressive and self-injurious. In any other environment for adults with disabilities, Don would not have the same quality of life he is able to maintain at Bittersweet Farms.

Victor

Reason for Admission

Victor's parents were not able to keep Victor at home because of his aggression and need for a structured environment. His behavioral episodes were frequent and extreme.

Background Information and History

Victor's parents moved to Ohio in order to place Victor at Bittersweet Farms. His parent chose Bittersweet because it was a farm and Victor is much calmer in nature. He resisted closed, restricted classrooms, and his parents felt that a farmstead model would provide a greater quality of life for him. Victor is deaf and had intensive sign language training since he was a young child. He was educated at a residential school for the deaf from ages 5 to 16 because there were no local programs where his parents lived.

The school worked in partnership with a program for children and adolescents with autism. In his mid-teens, Victor was flown to Connecticut and was admitted to another residential program specializing in autism. Victor is deaf, visually impaired, and has a moderate intellectual disability, although he tested in the gifted range as a young child. Victor has significant sensory processing deficits. Victor communicates with a basic repertoire of sign language. Victor was not on any medication when he was admitted to Bittersweet in 1986 at the age of 18. Since 2020, after the pandemic started, Victor has not been part of the Bittersweet program. He is currently living in a group home in the community and has not found a successful day program. The programs he has tried to attend have been traditional settings indoors which are not suited to Victor and an outdoor nature program has not been found. His parents are waiting to hear if Bittersweet has an opening for him again in the day program.

Main Problem

After his placement at Bittersweet, Victor developed pica. He would attempt to eat cigarette butts, brown paper towels, latex gloves, and cellophane. He also started chewing on his wooden bed frame. His pica resulted in bowel obstructions, and he had one major surgery to remove part of his colon. He had additional exploratory surgery to remove three to five latex gloves which had solidified and caused a blockage and a perforation. Because of the extreme danger of pica behavior, Victor required 24-hour, line-of-sight supervision. Victor was aggressive and severely bit his fingers and arms. He repeatedly hit himself in the head and legs. He could become physically aggressive toward others and hit, bite, push, and throw objects. Victor's physical aggression occurred when he was agitated or when he was redirected from pica consumption, but it could also occur when he was in good spirits.

Unique Approaches and Interventions

Victor's pica behaviors were challenging both to redirect or modify. He did respond to positive incentives or losing privileges. The best deterrent was to modify all environments. While Victor lived in the residence, he had an alarm on his door and on the door of the residential wing. He had close supervision while still allowing personal space. The staff visually swept the space on the farm and in the community during outings to remove cigarette butts and other targeted items. There were a series of guidelines and scripts for Victor to distract him from temptation. His limited communication and aggressive outbursts further complicated the situation. On community outings, when Victor would exit the vehicle, he was taken by the hand and reminded that if he was good, he could have a pop. If he began to look around the ground, he would be signed to keep his eyes up. He needed to be monitored in the public bathrooms and was usually compliant if he knew he was being watched. Victor was praised any time he passed through an area with a high concentration of objects. If Victor was searching for objects and dashed from staff, refusing to hold a staff member's hand, the staff would put themselves physically in Victor's path to block him from the object he was trying to get. The staff continued doing this until Victor cooperated and took their hand. Again, if Victor started looking for objects, he was signed to look up and praised for any self-restraint. If Victor obtained an object and ingested it, there were medical protocols to follow, and he could have been taken to the emergency room.

Interventions for Victor's aggressive behaviors were varied. Exercise was always important for Victor, and the intensive hiking schedule and gross motor work activities helped him. If he was aggressive, he was taken for a two-mile hike to calm down. Hiking and working in the woods provided Victor with the proprioceptive input he needed to remain calm. Victor did best when working with male staff who liked to be outdoors. Victor could be engaged by hauling firewood, cleaning up brush, and doing other big heavy gross motor activities which provided the sensory input he so desperately needed. Victor could be easily overstimulated. For example, Detroit Redwings tickets were donated to Bittersweet and Victor and several other residents attended. After 15 minutes, Victor was in such a state of sensory overload that the group had to leave. Victor would have been better off out in nature with activities which provided the sensory input he needed!

Additional behavioral interventions were developed that included asking Victor to explain what upset him and help him relax. If Victor wanted more space, staff took him away from others or depopulated the area. The staff always explained when a task was going to be finished and praised him for calming down. Victor preferred working with men who took the time to establish a rapport with him. This became a problem with the high turnover of staff. Additionally, as the residents aged, activities had to be modified and did not adequately support Victor's sensory system. Other residents could be in aerobic activities by being in sports, but Victor was too violent to participate in the Special Olympic teams. If Victor was self-injurious or aggressive toward others, other staff were asked to provide assistance.

In later years, medication was used to help control his behavior. In 2004, Victor was transferred to a local more restrictive setting after the annual state review found him too aggressive and the Bittersweet staff were unable to provide adequate support. This facility has a medical clinic with a nurse, psychiatrist, psychologist, and a behavior support expert who is more experienced with aggressive and violent behaviors. Victor's medications were reviewed and reduced, and a behavior plan was developed. After three months, Victor returned to Bittersweet to participate in the day program, Monday through Friday, between 8.30 am and 3.00 pm. During the pandemic in 2020, the day program was temporarily closed.

Quality-of-Life Changes

Victor made substantial changes in six of the eight QOL domains. Victor's problematic behaviors remained severe, but his quality-of-life evaluation indicates that he has made substantial gains in his QOL. In the domain of emotional well-being, Victor made substantial progress in contentment (satisfaction, moods, enjoyment). He had much less stress being in a rural setting with outdoor activities. Being out in nature, particularly the woods, calmed him down. In the domain of self-determination, Victor made minimal progress in developing independence. He had to be closely supervised because of his pica and his aggression. He was unable to develop personal control of his behaviors. However, Victor responded, like other residents, to the structure of the day and the flexibility of various activities, which gave him choices. Victor had developed more social interactions and relationships in the Bittersweet program. He made gains in the domains of interpersonal relations and social inclusion. Victor enjoyed his space and preferred to be by himself, but when he had a strong relationship with a staff member, he intermittently engaged in reciprocal activities. Victor enjoyed the activities on the farm but also seemed to benefit therapeutically from activities in the community. Victor enjoyed outings but these outings had to be limited because of his high propensity for pica in any uncontrolled environment. Although Victor's activities were limited by his behaviors, he had a much greater quality of life at Bittersweet than he currently has in a group home attending indoor classrooms and workshops.

Discussion

Victor responded to the peacefulness of the farm and the outdoor activities. When he was a young adult, if he became aggressive, a two-mile hike through the woods would calm him down. He liked working in the woodshed and in gross motor activities which required him to lift, push, and pull, providing him with sensory input. He participated in landscaping and mowing the lawn. The emphasis on activity and aerobic exercise was beneficial for Victor, making the farmstead setting a far superior residential setting for him. Although Victor did not initiate interaction, he benefited from the partnership aspect of Bittersweet. A speech and language therapist worked intensively with Victor and helped the staff enhance his receptive and expressive communication. For example, Victor was encouraged to use a "reality board" for storytelling that defines the weather, temperature, lunch menu, notable activities of the day, and how he is feeling. Storytelling uses sign language and simple pictures. Victor was encouraged to expand the storylines into complete simple sentences or phrases. The staff were instructed to use sign language to describe activities and what was happening around the farm to help Victor understand his surroundings and anticipate what would be happening next. This speaks to the importance of a full-time speech therapist on staff!

Victor responded to the structure of the farm and the staff worked to keep him in a routine of hiking, eating with the group, and fully participating in activities. Victor's focus on activities and completing goals reduced his aggression and consumption of pica objects. Victor enjoyed cutting and stacking wood and clearing trails. Victor's parents observed at a young age that Victor was more peaceful and calmer in a rural setting. Bittersweet was the perfect placement for Victor to receive the benefits of nature and the sensory input of long hikes and hard physical work.

Gus

Reason for Admission

Gus was admitted to Bittersweet Farms in 1984 when he was 19 years old because his parents were no longer able to cope with his behavior. Gus was physically larger than his parents and was hitting and occasionally throwing objects. His parents were not able to provide him with the structure and support he needed, and they were developing health problems.

Background Information and History

Gus was the youngest of eight children and was diagnosed with autism as a preschooler. He received special education from preschool until high school graduation. At the time of placement, Gus exhibited behavior problems such as temper tantrums, rocking, withdrawal, and minimal verbal interactions with others. His interactions with others were related to trying to communicate his wants and needs. Gus was too anxious to participate in activities and would run in the front yard for an hour or more to calm down. He was aggressive at Bittersweet the way he was at home, and would do two-fisted hitting. This behavior is now rare. His rituals and compulsions were very rigid which interfered with his productivity. Gus could become very aggressive if his rituals were interrupted. Gus had a mild intellectual disability, limited expressive language, sensory processing deficits, and an obsessive-compulsive disorder.

Main Problem

Gus' main problem when he entered Bittersweet was aggression. His long-term goal was to eliminate aggression and to develop self-control. Gus would become agitated if corrected or upset about something before he could express himself. He could suddenly hit someone or something.

Unique Approaches and Interventions

An occupational therapy evaluation provided the staff with the information necessary to plan Gus' work and recreational activities which would calm him and reduce anxiety. In addition to the daily hikes, Gus was allowed to run for more than an hour to help him calm down. Hiking in the woods is better than walking on the track, as it requires using all the senses. It is necessary to walk carefully on the trail without tripping over rocks and tree roots and to plan how to avoid them. Hiking in the woods provides the sensory input Gus needs.

Gus was encouraged to do weaving, use a push mower to mow the lawn, engage in other pushing and pulling activities, and do other chores on the farm that require the use of both upper extremities. He was encouraged to use the swing or rocking chair to provide vestibular input when he became upset or agitated. Activities which provided a variety of tactile sensations provided proprioceptive input. Sensory-based interventions provided Gus with a means of calming himself. Additional interventions for aggression consisted of many preventive techniques used by the staff. For example, they inform Gus of the schedule each day and evening at the beginning of each shift. They give explanations and suggestions rather than "orders," and they give corrections in an indirect manner. Gus is encouraged to verbalize his feelings and frustrations. If Gus appears anxious, the staff try to find out what is bothering him and help him problem solve. If Gus wants to run to calm himself, the staff encourage him to first complete a portion of the task in which he is involved so that running does not become an avoidance technique.

In 1987, Gus had a medication change because he was suddenly hitting and could not express his frustration appropriately. He might hit the person nearest to him, even if that person was not involved. In 1988, Gus was given relaxation exercises to help him relax when he became extremely tense. He was taught deep breathing exercises which, despite becoming ritualized, helped him. These exercises were practiced three to seven times a week for approximately 15–30 minutes. He was also encouraged to walk around the farm to become calm. Daily behavior sheets recorded Gus' mild and severe agitation, hitting, and repetitive hitting. These monthly records indicated that Gus' behavior in 1989 involved between 16 and 17 incidents of mild agitation, and 1 or 2 incidents of severe agitation. He rarely engaged in hitting. In 1990, Gus became more agitated with 28 incidents of mild agitation and 4 incidents of severe agitation occurring in February. Over the next few months, between 21 incidents of mild agitation and 7 incidents of severe agitation were calculated. Severe agitation dropped and he rarely hit anyone.

During 1991 and 1992, Gus' frequency of mild agitation dropped considerably to between nine and five times a month with no incidents of hitting. In 1992, Gus was away from the farm for six months for cancer treatment. A psychology report indicated that in 1993, Gus was less aggressive and still responded well to structure and consistency in his environment. In 2004, it was reported that Gus was not aggressive and actually became anxious if others around him were aggressive or displaying maladaptive behaviors. Gus' aggression was rated as severe when he entered Bittersweet and is currently viewed as mild by the staff.

Quality-of-Life Changes

Gus had a limited quality of life when he arrived at Bittersweet, but over time, he improved in all eight QOL domains. His unpredictable and sudden hitting made it difficult to take him into public settings. His independence was limited, and he had no specific skills. He had difficulty with self-care skills and limited interaction with others. Gus has made substantial gains in the emotional well-being domain. He has learned to be productive through the years in horticulture therapy, gardening, and crafting. When the art program was started, Gus found his home as a creative artist. His paintings are in demand and sell first during shows. He is content and feels proud of his accomplishments and his activities give him purpose and enjoyment. Gus is no longer socially isolated.

Gus has gained substantial progress in the domains of interpersonal relations and social inclusion. He is supported in the Bittersweet community and has people with whom he is comfortable. He now enjoys many community activities, such as shopping, movies, art exhibits, and eating out. In the domain of personal development, Gus has developed art skills and paints pictures on commission for people in the area. He also sells his pictures at Bittersweet in the gift shop. In the domain of self-determination, Gus is independent around the farm, completes his goals, and is given many choices. Gus has made significant improvement in all areas of quality-of-life domains, and within the Bittersweet context, has no problems in most areas.

Discussion

The farmstead model provided the structured programming that Gus needed to reduce his anxiety and to develop prevocational skills. Purposeful activities, such as working with animals, have helped Gus to focus his attention outside himself. Recreational programs and social games with turn taking increased his awareness of others. All the activities are done in partnership with the staff and have allowed Gus to develop relationships and increase his communication skills. Speech and language interventions were developed for the staff to help Gus express his feelings, voice his wants and needs, and communicate on a broader scale. When Gus came to Bittersweet, he needed to run to become calm when agitated. Often, he would run for an hour or more in the front yard. He has profited from the active recreational program of hiking, sports, and the Special Olympics. The farm setting, with long distances to walk and physical chores to complete, such as taking care of the animals and maintaining the property, has helped Gus reduce his anxiety by meeting his sensory needs. During his free time, Gus walks miles around the track each day. As Gus became more independent and his self-help skills increased, he moved into co-op housing with five other male residents and participates in cooking and cleaning. He enjoys more independence and can tolerate his housemates. Gus is an introvert and prefers quiet areas. He is protective of the arm that had cancer and reconstructive surgery. He will remove himself from an area he does not care for. The farmstead allows him the ability to have the peace and quiet that soothes him. A group home with traditional activities in a workshop or in an indoor area for crafts would not allow Gus to receive the sensory input and aerobic activities to address his aggression and anxiety. Without activities tailored to his sensory needs, Gus would not have been able to increase his quality of life.

Ian

Reason for Admission

Ian's mother wanted him to reach his highest potential in a humane environment.

Background Information and History

Ian attended special education classes through high school and had a positive attitude toward his teachers and school. He was independent in his self-care and could dress and undress himself, toilet himself, and eat independently. Ian exhibited many behaviors consistent with his diagnosis of autism and mild intellectual disability. He lacked awareness of others and had a severely impaired ability to make peer friendships. He was generally withdrawn, had poor eye contact, and would sit for long periods of time staring. He had a lack of community safety skills, and his language skills were impacted by his verbal perseveration. Ian had a restricted range of interests and was usually preoccupied with listening to his music. He had never been aggressive but could become inappropriately fidgety and giggly. Ian became distressed over changes to his routine. Ian was 23 years old when he was admitted to Bittersweet in 1986.

Main Problem

Ian's greatest problem at the time of his admission was his tendency to withdraw. He had extreme difficulty remaining on task without continual staff supervision, including tasks he knew how to perform. There seemed to be no clear pattern or cause attached to his withdrawal, but this behavior interfered with Ian's ability to be independent, productive, and integrate into the Bittersweet community. Consequently, Ian had poor relationships with his peers and had difficulty focusing on all aspects of his daily life.

Unique Approaches and Interventions

Bittersweet focused on Ian's tendency to withdraw from his environment and individuals. A plan was put in place to have him participate in vigorous activities, which required attention in order to participate, such as tennis, baseball, and volleyball. Vocationally, he was placed in activities which required large motor skills, such as horticulture and animal care, which would help him focus his attention and receive sensory input. The staff was instructed to find two or three tasks that Ian had already mastered and needed little direction to complete. Ian was shown all the steps in the task. If he became distracted or withdrew from the task in other ways, he was redirected and praised when the task was completed. This strategy encouraged interaction and communication with the staff. Ian was then paired with another resident, who could also complete the same task and Ian was asked to be the "teacher" and work alongside the person to help when necessary. This was designed to help Ian feel a sense of responsibility and success, which hopefully would provide motivation. Ian has been able to live in a co-op house which has helped him be less withdrawn. The men share responsibilities for the care of the house, such as cooking and cleaning. As a group, they plan activities such as going to the movies or the pool, or choosing videos. This small community in the co-op has helped Ian stay interactive and has allowed him to develop friendships. His treatment plan to reduce his withdrawal was met in September 1999.

Quality-of-Life Changes

Ian made substantial improvement in all eight QOL domains. Ian entered the Bittersweet program generally withdrawn, sitting for long periods of time staring. His lack of awareness of others significantly impaired his ability to make friends. He was moderately anxious, depressed, and withdrawn. Ian has made substantial gains in the domains of interpersonal relations and social inclusion. He is no longer anxious or depressed and only mildly withdrawn. As Ian has become less withdrawn, his interaction with others and his awareness of his environment have greatly increased his quality of life. He loves being active and has participated in the Special Olympics in tennis, flying to the 2000 Nationals with a group of other Special Olympians. He is much more interactive and greets people coming to the farm.

Ian has made substantial improvement in the domain of personal development. He likes the farm and enjoys groundskeeping, using the mower, and working in the horticulture program. He has now achieved the status of excelling in sports, especially for his awards in tennis. In the domain of self-determination, he has choices and is very independent at the farm. He is able to be productive and reach his goals at work. He is able to go on vacations with his mother to Paris and Hawaii.

Discussion

The Bittersweet model that emphasizes community interaction, partnership, structure, and aerobic activity has been the perfect environment for Ian. It has allowed him to transform over the years to the quality of life which he currently enjoys. All of the above-mentioned aspects of the Bittersweet program have been important in encouraging Ian to become less withdrawn, to develop friendships, to exercise better interactive skills, and to experience a sense of responsibility and motivation. The farmstead setting with its large motor activities and physical activity gives him the opportunity to engage in work he finds fulfilling, such as groundskeeping, mowing, and horticulture. The farm activities also provide him with the sensory input he needs. Ian had previously failed in a workshop setting. The workshop setting would not have provided Ian with the sensory input, social communication, and partnership he needed and would not have encouraged him to be less withdrawn. Ian has and continues to benefit from the predictable structure of the farmstead. He finds the routine calming, as do most of the residents. Because Ian is now an integral part of the farm community, he is motivated to vary his schedule and go on outings. The turn taking nature of sports such as tennis, baseball, and volleyball has helped Ian to focus on others and stay on task. The activities also provide a social group and interaction with others. Working in partnership with the staff provided Ian with opportunities to increase his communication skills. Ian still requires supervision because he has no safety insight and still has difficulty staying on task. For example, once while cooking, he stepped away from the stove, and his grilled cheese sandwich burned. During a 911 class, he stepped over the body, missing the key understanding of the lesson. Not being able to show judgment in these situations makes his behavior a safety risk.

Interview Notes

During an interview on October 28, 2020, when asked what he liked best about Bittersweet, Ian indicated that he liked mowing the grass. "When I use the riding mower," he said, "I like relaxing and seeing what I'm doing. I got a job out in the community working at One Source, mowing the grass and janitorial." When asked what he does with the money, Ian said that he buys new stuff. Ian was asked if there was anything he didn't like about the farm. His response: "I like the farm. Being outdoors and indoors. Everything."

Jon

Reason for Admission

Jon was aggressive, and his parents were unable to control him.

Background Information and History

Before Jon moved to Bittersweet, he had a history of severe behavior problems. Jon had a psychotic break during 1974 and 1975, requiring hospitalization, after which he was placed in a residential treatment center between ages 10 and 13. When Jon was 17 years old and still in a structured school program, his behavior escalated and he started to be physically hostile to his father, slapping, spitting at him, and hitting him. The family could not restrain him, and Jon was heavily medicated in an effort to control him. During this difficult time, Jon's parents looked for help and were turned down because of lack of appropriate placements. One day, before his medication took effect, Jon attacked his father and the police were called to help restrain him. The police suggested that if this continued, the family should take him to a long-term psychiatric hospital.

Jon was 20 years old when he came to Bittersweet in 1983. He was obsessed with calling his father and shouting ritualistic phrases and stories. He was often aggressive, pushing people to get to the phone. If the staff intervened, he would become aggressive. He had inappropriate sexual behaviors and obsessions, destroyed property, and took money and objects he needed for his projects, such as scotch tape and scissors. He would perseverate on inanimate objects such as vacuum cleaners, elevators, and escalators. His interaction with the staff was limited to his wants and needs and most of his language was ritualistic. Jon had moderate expressive and receptive language skills and a mild intellectual disability. Jon was severely withdrawn and anxious and had sensory integration deficits.

Main Problem

Jon's main problem when he came to Bittersweet was his inappropriate sexual behavior. He would expose himself and masturbate in public when he became agitated. He would smell women inappropriately and smell places where women had been sitting. Jon is hypersensitive to olfactory input and has an active response which drives him to do very inappropriate behaviors. He was fixated on the color red and would get under red cars and masturbate.

Unique Approaches and Interventions

Jon's inappropriate sexual behaviors were connected to his agitation and anxiety. Incorporating Jon into the structure at the farm and establishing relationships with the staff through partnership activities were the first steps in his intervention. Jon responded to the structure at the farm and the constant supervision and became less anxious. Initially, he began participating in the horticulture department at the prevocational level, learning farm life skills. Over time, the daily schedule of work in partnership with staff helped reduce his anxiety as he learned new skills, became more focused on activities, and his communication skills improved with interaction. To help Jon reduce his anxiety, he was also scheduled for vigorous exercise three times a week. Jon was involved in work that was physical in nature and therefore calming, as it provided sensory input. Jon mowed the lawn with a hand mower, cut wood with a two-person saw, and was in the horticulture department digging, hauling, and lifting—all of which provided vigorous exercise. Jon was also on the Special Olympics swim team. In addition, Jon participated in two- to three-mile hikes after work each day and a Saturday hike of five to six miles.

Jon received two hours of counseling a week to help him understand his behavior choices and how his behavior affected others. Counseling was also used to increase his language and communication skills. Jon arrived at Bittersweet in 1983 and staff notes indicate that in 1987 Jon was engaging in inappropriate sexual behaviors one to three times a week and would run through the house yelling and demanding to call his father to repeat ritualistic conversations. He was still resisting farm and community activities approximately six times a day. He did this by locking himself in a room and insisting he could not participate. To reduce anxiety, a predictable year-long family visit schedule was planned. This included phone calls to his family twice a week. The staff continued to involve Jon in a full schedule of meaningful farm, home, and community activities under constant supervision. Behavior plans were developed in 1989 to help eliminate Jon's inappropriate sexual behavior. After three months, there was a noticeable decrease in his inappropriate sexual behaviors. His 1990 annual psychology review indicated that these behaviors were reduced to 3 in the previous three months, down from 15 incidents per month the previous year. In 1990, Jon had a behavioral goal to not touch women, feel their arms, or smell them. A cue was developed to have him back up an arm's length from people. A nurse met with him regularly along with the psychology assistant to role play appropriate sexual behavior. Jon's annual assessments in 1992 and 1993 indicated that there were no incidents of sexual behaviors. However, Jon continued to have aggressive behaviors and severe agitation that resulted in other behavioral problems. His sexual behaviors are now so infrequent that they are not charted.

Quality-of-Life Changes

Jon made substantial improvement in all eight domains of quality of life. In the domain of emotional well-being, Jon became more a part of the Bittersweet community. Eliminating the inappropriate sexual behaviors made this integration into the community possible. He then found activities and jobs at which he excelled. Jon is now more content and less anxious. Accomplishing productive work allows Jon to experience a sense of self-worth. Improvement in the domain of material well-being is reflected in Jon's work in the kitchen. For this, he earns minimum wage, which he can spend as he pleases. Improvement in the domains of interpersonal relations and social inclusion is reflected in Jon's relationships with his peers, staff, and family—all of which have improved significantly. Jon also receives support in his work environment. Now that Jon is no longer aggressive, he can enjoy a variety of leisure activities. He enjoys swimming at the Y, going to church, and hiking every day. Within the structure of Bittersweet and the staff support, Jon enjoys an excellent quality of life. Just ask him!

Discussion

The Bittersweet farmstead model was critical for Jon. He came to the farm isolated, aggressive, and lacked interaction with others. The daily work schedule, with purposeful activities, motivated him to become involved with people. Farm activities, which required him to lift, carry, walk, and engage in physical activities, helped reduce his anxiety by providing him with sensory input. He participated in the daily hikes and the Saturday extended hike. Among the many tasks on the farm, Jon found activities he was interested in and where he experienced success. He enjoyed the status of being an expert in using the rototiller, for example. Another setting that did not require physical activity would not have been as calming. The emphasis on aerobic activities and the Special Olympics helped Jon stabilize his emotions. Jon was given guitar lessons, and he played in the hand bell choir. Jon found a place in a community, and his aggression and obsessive behaviors lessened as his interactive skills improved. He found a sense of self-worth as his talents became more evident. Currently, Jon enjoys working in the kitchen and the horticulture and art programs. Jon, like many residents, has cycled through periods of productivity and times of behavioral disruption. In another work setting, he would have lost his job and become isolated from his community. At Bittersweet, job adjustments were made while he was being evaluated and helped to stabilize. After that, he could return to the job settings where he felt successful again. Jon continues to need the consistent structure of Bittersweet and help to control and reduce his maladaptive behaviors.

Interview Notes

Jon was interviewed on March 30, 2011. He said that life was going very good! He was happy that the staff help him set goals. He wants to be a waiter at the Whitehouse Inn and save money to buy a house in Whitehouse. He likes his options and choices. He likes to listen to music, ride bikes, and work in the art room, workshop, kitchen, and horticulture areas. Jon was interviewed again on October 28, 2020. When asked what he liked about Bittersweet, he said the co-op house, because he has roommates and he named all of them. He said he likes to watch movies in his bedroom and listen to music. He also liked to be outside on the farm, mostly swimming on a hot day in the summertime. He hikes twice around the track on Mondays through Fridays which is a quarter mile. Jon was asked if he would have liked to have lived in Cleveland, where he is from. He responded by saying that he didn't like rushing around every day in the city and getting heart attacks and riding the buses and wearing his shoes out. Living at Bittersweet gets him away from the congestion of the city. He said he is a "Country Gentleman Farmer!"

Ken

Reason for Admission

Ken was admitted to Bittersweet in 1983. He had been in the foster care system and required a group home placement.

Background Information and History

Ken fell from a balcony at the age of two, after which his development severely regressed. Diagnoses of infantile autism, retardation, and brain damage were noted in previous psychological tests. Protective services gained custody of Ken when he was four years old, and he was placed in a foster home. Ken remained in the foster care system until he was placed at Bittersweet Farms, where he had been in the day program while in high school.

Ken has a mild intellectual disability and severe communication problems. At the time of admission, Ken had an oral reading score at the sixth-grade level, reading comprehension at the fourth-grade level, spelling at the ninth-grade level, and math computation at the third-grade level. Ken was not overly communicative and much of his language was echolalic. He exhibited some bizarre stereotypic behavior and lacked good eye contact. He has sensory processing deficits.

Main Problem

A psychological report in 1988 indicated that Ken had developed some aggressive behaviors. He pushed a resident and staff member after being asked to make a transition to a new task. The staff felt that Ken was stimulated by other residents' acting out behavior and may have been imitating them. He exhibited self-injurious behavior and withdrawal.

Unique Approaches and Interventions

Ken's aggressive behaviors occur in both recreational and vocational settings. He is sensitive to the words "no" and "please." If the staff use a voice inflection indicative of correction, Ken will frequently have an outburst. Ken's sensory processing deficits are addressed by hiking and working in areas that require physical activity. These activities provide him with the proprioceptive input he needs. In 2005, Ken experienced an almost constant level of agitation that had not been seen before. New residential housing was being built, and he indicated that he would like to go back to the time before the construction. The structure of the farm is important for Ken as evidenced by his emotional upset when changes occur. In 1990, Ken was moved to the co-op house with a smaller number of residents and seemed to enjoy the company and the group activities. Ken gets on well with the staff and other residents, and he enjoys his vocational placements. Currently, Ken has a goal of decreasing episodes of being upset to no more than twice a month. The staff are encouraged to cue Ken to take some deep breaths, engage in a different task, or leave the area to a safe place. They encourage him to communicate why he is upset but not press him to answer. They may suggest that he write down what is upsetting him. The staff assist Ken in finding preferred and meaningful activities. The same interventions are used when Ken does self-injurious behaviors, which occur six or seven times a month. Physical aggression occurs more than three times a month. Similar interventions are used.

Quality-of-Life Changes

Ken has improved substantially in all eight quality-of-life domains. In the domain of social inclusion, Ken is involved in the community as a participant in activities and as a volunteer. He likes participating in Special Olympic sporting events and practices. He also enjoys going to the library, especially a popular culture library at a neighboring university. He goes with a group of residents to a local church on Sundays and enjoys shopping and going out to dinner. When a job was available at a local pizzeria, he did janitorial work and kitchen preparation. He was able to visit the Outer Banks in North Carolina in 2018. In the domain of self-determination, he has a great deal of independence and many choices and options of activities. As long as Ken notifies the staff of his whereabouts beforehand, he is able to move safely on the Bittersweet grounds unsupervised by staff with a visual check every 30 minutes. Ken needs minimal support on established tasks, and is a good worker. He must be supervised in the community with reminders by the staff of the safety rules, such as looking out for cars. In the domain of personal development, Ken has developed skills and made substantial gains in achievement and productivity.

Currently, Ken is involved in the following work activities: culinary, weaving, gardens, and art instruction. At times, he engages in a number of volunteer opportunities in the community. He is interested in possible opportunities for competitive employment in the community. In the domain of interpersonal relations, Ken has limited contact with his siblings, and his parents are deceased. Some employees of Bittersweet remain close to Ken and often include him in their homes for the holidays or whenever desired. Ken has limited communication skills which impacts his ability to be involved with peers and others, but he enjoys being part of group activities. Ken is friendly and likes to greet others. He is interested in learning people's names. He often asks questions of others but may not always respond when a question is directed at him. Ken's quality of life has increased dramatically since he arrived at Bittersweet. Despite his communication deficits, he now has friendships and "family" experiences with staff. He can remain calm because of the structure and be productive at the farm and in the community. He is his own guardian and makes choices in all areas of his life. He is allowed to be as independent as possible within the Bittersweet complex.

Discussion

The structure of the farm has helped Ken remain calm, allowing him to be productive in meaningful jobs at both the farm and in the community. The staff understand Ken's triggers, and they approach him in respectful ways that give him dignity. The partnership with staff has given him a sense of community and family. In traditional residential settings, there is usually a mix of people of different developmental problems, and the staff are not extensively trained in autism. It is the understanding of Ken's needs that has allowed Ken to obtain a high quality of life. The active life at Bittersweet helps Ken with his ever-present anxiety. He is involved in landscaping and other tasks which keep him outdoors and moving. He benefits from hiking, which provides him with multisensory input. He has difficulty making eye contact easily and hiking activates his visual system to keep him from running into trees. This active, outdoor life increases Ken's quality of life. A more traditional residential model could not provide this important element.

Interview Notes

In an interview on October 28, 2020, Ken indicated that he likes bowling and washing dishes. He also likes living on a farm and asked about when former staff members were going to visit. He likes being outside, especially raking leaves and drinking coffee outdoors.

Larry

Reason for Admission

Larry lived with his parents until he was 13 years old, at which time he was placed in a group home. Larry had developed aggressive behaviors, and these behaviors were interfering with his family's ability to function. In 1983, when Larry turned 18 years old, he was placed at Bittersweet Farms.

Background Information and History

Larry is the oldest of four children and, other than pneumonia at one month old, he had an unremarkable medical history. He attended classes for the intellectually disabled and graduated from a multi-handicapped classroom. Larry was described as being a low functioning autistic. He has moderate intellectual deficit and did not attend well to tasks. He had poor eating habits without constant monitoring. Larry had limited verbal expression but had good receptive language skills and was able to follow two-step directions. Larry was able to speak, but it often took prompting. He has poor articulation. Larry has sensory processing deficits and an obsessive-compulsive disorder.

Main Problem

Aggression was Larry's major problem when he started at Bittersweet. He would throw things, scream, yell, run, and repetitively say, "Last chance, ask Grandma." Once he picked up a bike and threw it at a car. He would yell constantly for hours and plug toilets every time he had a chance. These were severe and disruptive behaviors which were costly because of the bathroom flooding continually.. Larry would have daily outbursts when he arrived.

Unique Approaches and Interventions

A thorough occupational therapy evaluation indicated that Larry had difficulty filtering or modifying sensory information, was under-registering sensation—especially vestibular and proprioceptive sensations—and demonstrated exaggerated emotional responses to sensory events. The evaluation suggested the following activities:

1. Provide a fast brushing and joint compression exercise routine three times per day. This can also be used during early signs of agitation.

2. When riding a moving piece of equipment on hikes or when riding his bike, provide Larry with uneven vestibular stimulation, i.e., jerky, bumpy roads/trails, etc., so that he needs to co-contract his muscles.
3. During Larry's normal daily routines, provide him with opportunities that require gross motor movement and physical activity. Ask Larry to help with activities that involve pushing, pulling, carrying, and lifting. These suggestions will provide Larry with the proprioceptive/kinesthetic feedback that he requires. These activities are also physical and high energy and may assist with decreasing some of Larry's aggressive behaviors.
4. Encourage Larry to participate in weaving at least five days a week. This occupation will provide him with proprioceptive/kinesthetic feedback through joint compression as well as tactile sensation.

When Larry entered Bittersweet, he was placed in the farmworker program to meet his needs for vigorous physical activity and gross motor tasks which gave him the sensory input he needed. He engaged in a combination of routine barn tasks and seasonal outdoor activities, such as gardening, orchard, and woodland work. Larry was also included in hiking, biking, and swimming lessons. He enjoyed playing in the pool. All of these activities provided the sensory input Larry needed to remain emotionally stable.

A farmstead is a perfect setting for residents with significant sensory deficits. Farm tasks which require heavy lifting, pushing, and pulling are excellent interventions. In order to increase Larry's awareness of others, he was included in community activities, such as going to restaurants, roller skating, and movies. He was also involved in small-group activities where he and another resident would be required to communicate and share responsibility to complete a task. In 1991, a psychological report indicated that Larry was resistant to being involved in the program and his vocational placement. For hours at a time, Larry would sit on the ground and rock, refusing to participate in any activity offered, while screaming himself hoarse. On several occasions, Larry would spend days sitting on the ground, yelling, and not wanting to do anything. Behavioral programs were unsuccessful. This was attributed to Larry's low IQ score and his inability to generalize learning, which is common with people with autism.

Vocationally, Larry continued to be inflexible in his ability to transfer from one area to another. In 1994, it was reported that Larry would spend 10–20 hours a month yelling which took up much staff time and was disruptive to the other participants. The staff were concerned over

Larry's increased yelling and resistance to be involved with the program. He needed intense behavior management and structure to maintain continued progress toward independence. He needed monthly reviews for his psychotropic medication.

Bittersweet allows Larry to choose work which meets his need for sensory stimulation. He loves cutting wood as compared to trying to sand a piece of wood evenly. Larry usually ends up sanding a groove in one spot. Larry can cut wood for hours! In 1994, it was decided that Larry would do better in a sheltered workshop with repetitive tasks, which seemed to agree with him. He spent over 15 years attending a workshop during the day. When the project ended and Larry returned to the Bittersweet day program, his behaviors escalated.

To help Larry when he's withdrawn, staff encourage him to choose from a variety of activities. His preferences are noted on a schedule with pictures and/or short and direct written instructions. The schedule is reviewed with him throughout the day. Larry is encouraged to be active and is given positive attention. The staff explain the benefits and purpose of the activities to help motivate him. In 2003, Larry had 12 documented occasions of self-injurious behaviors in the past year and then none over the next three months. When Larry is physically aggressive, staff are encouraged to back away and give Larry his space. The staff will not emotionally or negatively react through their words, tone, or body language. They will block his kicks, hits, or thrown items with crossed arms and open palms or use a soft cushion or blocking pad to absorb any force. Behavioral interventions included helping Larry verbalize his feelings of anger with appropriate words and volume. A quiet environment seems to help Larry relax. Larry can be asked to take a walk with staff and told that he is in a safe place. The staff are encouraged to talk about Larry's interest in Star Wars and Batman, give him compliments, explain reasons behind requests, and always review expectations.

Quality-of-Life Changes

Larry made substantial changes in five of the eight quality-of-life indicators. Larry was admitted to Bittersweet with severe anxiety, obsessive/compulsive behaviors, aggression, and self-injurious behaviors. He was severely withdrawn and had psychotic symptoms. After more than 35 years, Larry still has severe anxiety and obsessive-compulsive behaviors but has shown some improvement in aggression and self-injurious behavior. Yet, despite Larry's complex problems, he has made great gains in his quality of life within the Bittersweet environment. In the domains of interpersonal relations and social inclusion, Larry has made substantial gains as a result of the Bittersweet structure. He is given emotional support and participates in group activities. He has developed relationships with staff members. Because Larry's behavior has improved, he participates in community activities and averages about six outings per month—mostly for shopping, swimming, church, library, and walking in various parks. He usually attends summer camping trips and fairs when offered. He has a community of friends.

Larry has made some progress in the domains of personal development and self-determination. He has resisted participating in work activities and has not achieved independence, although he is given many choices. Larry still has continuous supervision at Bittersweet. He may spend some time alone, but staff will get a visual check on him every few minutes. He enjoys magazines/catalogs, shooting basketball hoops, playing catch, dining out, watching movies (Star Wars, science fiction), and being engaged in hands-on tasks. Larry enjoys walking around the track, which has become a ritual. He does not like to participate in sports, but loves going to baseball games. Larry's preferences for activities are those which give him sensory input. He likes to run his hands through puzzle pieces and sit with a weighted vest on his lap. Larry is given choices of activities and allowed to work in situations which give him needed sensory input.

Discussion

The structure and support at Bittersweet helped Larry understand the world around him. The consistency, expectations, guidelines, and choices helped Larry reduce his anxiety. As the years have passed, Larry has become comfortable with his life and is less upset. Larry has profited from the partnership aspect of the Bittersweet model, which is not part of a traditional model where staff are more supervisors. He has limited awareness of others but has developed some strong relationships with the staff. These relationships have added greatly to his quality of life. Larry often shares jokes or teasing interactions which give him pleasure as evidenced by his smile. Larry was even included in a staff member's wedding!

Bittersweet allows Larry to participate in large motor activities throughout the farm. These activities are critical in giving him the sensory input he needs to be calm. Farm activities involve heavy work, such as cutting the grass with an old-fashioned push mower, pushing a heavy wheelbarrow, cutting wood, and hauling it back to the farm. These are not activities of a traditional residential center for the severely disabled. The farmstead provides the sensory stimulation Larry and the other residents need to remain calm. The farm gives Larry 80 acres to walk, work, and be in nature, which he finds very calming when he is upset.

Norm

Reason for Admission

Norm's parents were unable to control his temper outbursts and could not manage his behavior. In 1985, Norm moved to a group home placement and did well, but his parents did not feel he could reach his potential. His parents felt that Bittersweet could help him develop a better quality of life within the limits of his disability. Norm was admitted to Bittersweet in 1987 at the age of 21.

Background Information and History

Norm is the third child in his family. His mother reported that he had a normal rate of development until about one year of age. The symptoms of his problems were first noted at 18 months, when Norm would cry for long periods of time and become indifferent to people and his environment. His speech was extremely delayed, and he did not begin using sentences until age 7. Norm has a mild intellectual disability and was in special education programs from when he was three years old. Norm has always had a special interest in numbers. For example, Norm is able to tell you the day of the week you were born on by your birth date and year. When Norm came to the farm, he had a significant obsessive-compulsive disorder and obsessions about time. He exhibited self-injurious and psychotic behaviors. Norm has sensory processing deficits and is hypersensitive to sounds. His speech was unrelated to what was being talked about at the time; and his expressive and receptive language skills were limited. He screamed when he was anxious and was aggressive toward others. He was shy and withdrawn and unable to socialize. His hyperactivity and inattention made it difficult to stay on task and be productive.

Main Problem

Norm had outbursts consisting of yelling, hitting himself, breathing hard, and screaming. He would also become aggressive if he was interrupted during his rituals. In the first 90 days of his placement at Bittersweet, Norm averaged seven outbursts per month.

Unique Approaches and Interventions

When Norm came to Bittersweet, he had so many frequent outbursts that he was unable to participate in community activities as well as family situations. He was hyperactive and without structure could not be productive. He was so withdrawn that he could not develop relationships. Eventually, Norm was moved to the co-op house and began doing chores with his housemates. Here, he began to develop a sense of community.

Giving Norm choices reduced his outbursts. He was given a great deal of structure but was free to decide which activities most interested him. Norm has many sensory problems. Recommendations for dealing with these sensory issues included encouraging him to swing or sit in a rocking chair and be involved in gross motor activities such as walking, hiking, and playing volleyball. Such activities were designed to have a calming effect on his nervous system.

Norm has difficulty in high stress situations, such as being in crowds and loud environments. His response includes running away and having an outburst. Norm's behavior support plans indicate that the staff could ask him if he would like to go outside if he is screaming indoors. He is encouraged to talk about what is bothering him. If there is a change in the schedule, Norm will be given advance notice, and if a task is too complex for him, the staff will break down the task into more manageable parts to reduce frustration. Norm's behavior is characterized by extreme aloneness, hypersensitivity to sound, and particular cognitive distortions, such as his unusual interest in numbers. His daily schedule includes walking to the entrance of the farm to get the daily paper. He is motivated to do this by his interest in statistics published in the paper, particularly in the sports section and lottery numbers. Norm rarely initiates conversation. He can be observed talking to himself about apparently irrelevant topics. Social interaction, such as the hand bell choir, and other group activities were recommended when he first came, to help him become more aware of others. Norm is encouraged to verbally communicate and express his desires, especially if he is leaving an area. Norm's ability to communicate his needs has improved. His speech is non-communicative but very interesting. For example, he might get upset and then say, "I'm sorry I violated my behavior support plan anyway" or "I'm still 21 percent upset!"

Quality-of-Life Changes

Norm made substantial gains in all eight of the QOL domains. In the domains of interpersonal relations and social inclusion, Norm made substantial progress as a result of the Bittersweet structure. Because Norm is withdrawn, his program includes discussion groups, outings, and team projects. He was also placed in a small housing unit of six persons, which allowed him to learn to cooperate with others. He is now able to participate in community outings, but still needs to be closely supervised because of his tendency to urinate in public.

Norm has made substantial gains in the domain of emotional wellbeing. The structure of the farm reduces the stress Norm felt in other settings. He feels content and experiences satisfaction in his activities. After Norm came to Bittersweet, he ran in a 10K race and continues to enjoy walking and hiking. Rather than play sports, he prefers to watch them. His parents take him to Tampa for baseball spring training, and Norm knows the names of the players and all their statistics. Norm is focused on the daily newspaper and can hardly wait to read the sports statistics. It has become his job to go to the end of the long driveway at the farm and pick up the paper each day. The paper is delivered at 4.30 am! Norm can be seen walking down the driveway in the dark with a flashlight!

Norm has made great gains in his quality of life after living and working at Bittersweet. Although he still has many areas of challenges, within the Bittersweet environment he no longer has problems that lead to aggression or severe anxiety. He has choices, hobbies, and vocational success at his level. The structure of the farm has been important to Norm. It reduces his anxiety and allows him to be productive. Interventions and supports—including structuring tasks for him—have helped him stay on task. Every aspect of the model has been important to Norm. While he's not motivated to do work, Norm can participate and knows he can take his time to complete a task. This flexibility might not be possible in a more traditional setting. Norm has benefited from the partnership aspect of the Bittersweet model. The staff have helped him work together with them and have encouraged more functional communication. Norm participates in all the activities and seems happy. The farmstead setting has been critical for Norm. He is calmer after he is outside doing sports or other activities which provide him with the sensory input he needs.

Interview Notes

During an interview on October 28, 2020, Norm was asked what he liked about Bittersweet. He said he liked to walk around the track a lot. He likes bowling and going out to eat. He gets to visit with his family. He likes living on a farm and working at the barn. Norm is good at numbers and is able to tell what day of the week someone was born on. He demonstrated that skill during the interview. He reads the sports pages and likes the Cleveland Browns and the Cleveland Indians. He likes working outdoors in the gardens. Norm said he couldn't think of anything to change about Bittersweet, and he liked it the way it is.

Oscar

Reason for Admission

Oscar was placed at Bittersweet Farms because his mother wanted a program that was structured and could provide Oscar with productive activities. She wanted him to continue and preserve the skills and opportunities Bette Ruth had provided Oscar in the Toledo public school setting. Oscar's father was sick, and his mother was exhausted taking care of both Oscar and his father. Oscar was diagnosed as autistic as a child and was in special education, both privately and in public school. He was a student of Bettye Ruth Kay in a high school multi-handicapped classroom.

Background Information and History

Oscar has an obsessive-compulsive disorder as well as autism. He has a mild intellectual disability. At the time of Oscar's admission, a speech therapy evaluation indicated that he had limited expressive language skills and that his vocabulary, both expressive and receptive, was at the five-year-old level. The content of his speech was very concrete. In spontaneous conversations, his responses were brief, and he did not take responsibility to maintain the conversation. Recommendations for increasing his language and communication skills were made which were then used by the staff in work and recreational settings. Oscar has sensory processing deficits.

When he was first placed at Bittersweet, Oscar worked at a structured workshop because he was experiencing success in that setting. His goals were for him to be as independent as possible. Oscar was admitted to Bittersweet in 1983 at the age of 25.

Main Problem

Oscar's extreme ritualistic behaviors interfered with his ability to function. If his rituals or compulsive behaviors were interrupted, he could be aggressive. When asked to do a task he did not enjoy, he would think nothing of being aggressive toward people or throwing heavy or dangerous objects at them.

Unique Approaches and Interventions

Oscar participated in specific vigorous seasonal physical activities to reduce stereotypic behavior and to maximize gross motor skills. The sensory input he received helped calm him down. He continues to enjoy heavy work such as lifting, pulling, and pushing, and hiking long distances. Oscar was placed in music therapy activities twice a week to increase his attention, awareness, and concentration and to decrease random and purposeless self-stimulating behavior. The staff took steps, which are still used, to prevent Oscar's physical aggression. The staff assist Oscar in developing a tangible, written schedule for the day, incorporating his choices and interests. They read Oscar's plan with him throughout the shift to ensure that he is prepared and that communication is consistent. Tasks are broken down into simple steps. The staff offer Oscar frequent breaks, especially when the environment is crowded. He is offered physical activity when he appears tense and frustrated. Oscar uses a boxing bag or a pillow to punch and he will engage in vigorous weaving and bread kneading for sensory input. He also uses cardio equipment as part of his activity plan. Oscar had problems with the change in seasons and how that affected what clothing he would wear. He was used to wearing long-sleeve shirts and, when the weather was very hot, the staff would have to be creative in helping him change his shirt after breakfast to a short-sleeve shirt. If the staff removed the long-sleeve shirt, he became aggressive. The staff developed consistent scripts that they would use at breakfast, "This is a very hot day. After you finish breakfast, you can hang your shirt back in the closet and wear a short-sleeve shirt." They would then question him and say, "What are you going to do after breakfast?" This was difficult for Oscar because he wanted to wear the same type of shirt each day and was frustrated with changes. Goals were set for Oscar to be able to communicate his needs and his emotions to enable him to tell staff his preferences in activities rather than acting impulsively. If Oscar became agitated, he was encouraged to walk around the track several times until he became calm. Autism and compulsive disorders are lifelong disabilities, and interventions cannot eliminate behaviors completely. Oscar, like other residents, continues to struggle with his behaviors. Oscar is aggressive between one and three times a month. His current annual goal is to reduce his physical aggression to an average of two or fewer incidents throughout the year.

Quality-of-Life Changes

Oscar has made significant gains in all eight quality-of-life domains. Oscar's quality of life was greatly improved by moving to Bittersweet

Farms. Living at home kept Oscar from forming relationships outside his family. Bittersweet's structure and its community-focused approach have increased Oscar's QOL in the domains of interpersonal relations and social inclusion. Oscar is now involved in recreational activities, travel, and community outings. Oscar's outings have included a trip to Chicago, wilderness camping, and backpacking. He enjoys going to the movies, roller skating, partaking in Special Olympic activities, swimming, and playing card games. Oscar has made substantial progress in the domains of personal development, physical well-being, and self-determination. He is continually taught individual self-help skills, such as doing his laundry and making nutritious lunches. He has developed skills in a variety of tasks on the farm and has shown growth in cooking, making bread, reading recipes, etc. He enjoys the many choices available to him and has some independence on the farm, although he is closely monitored to control some of his negative behaviors such as aggressive hugging when he is frustrated. Oscar is successful and productive.

Discussion

The active and aerobic nature of the farmstead model has been very important for Oscar. While Oscar continues to have difficulty expressing his emotions, physical activity helps him remain calm. All his behavior plans include engaging him in physical activity. Oscar enjoys downhill skiing, cross-country skiing, riding his bike and scooter around the track, and mountain climbing. He plays basketball, swims, and plays shuffleboard. He enjoys working with the animals. When he becomes agitated, he is encouraged to walk until he calms down. Oscar thrives on structure and consistency! The structure of the farm provides Oscar with the foundation he needs to understand his world and what is coming next during each day. The staff provide him with visual and verbal information about what is expected during the day. The spaciousness of the farm allows Oscar to move away from activities which are frustrating or cause him sensory problems.

The partnership component of the Bittersweet model is as critical for Oscar as it is for the other residents with severe autism, sensory issues, and compulsions. Each staff member assigned to Oscar understands how to work with him in a manner that helps prevent upsetting triggers. The communication and friendships that the staff develop with Oscar allow him to trust them and be motivated to complete tasks and be involved with new activities. Partnership also gives Oscar and the other residents a sense of community and awareness of the world around them. Oscar is popular with the staff, and he enjoys positive attention. He is developing a sense of humor. Oscar is part of the Bittersweet community and is included in social activities. The staff are aware of what triggers Oscar's stress and work to provide an environment that is relaxing and calm. Bittersweet is a community that promotes choices, independence, and purposeful activities. Within the structured and supportive environment of the farm, Oscar has made significant progress in all quality-of-life domains. The critical components which contributed to Oscar's progress can only be found on a farmstead. These components are not part of a traditional residential model.

Marvin

Reason for Admission

Marvin's parents thought that Bittersweet Farms could better meet his needs. He was admitted in 1985 when he was 20 years old.

Background Information and History

Marvin attended special education classes and lived at home before being admitted to Bittersweet Farms. He attended a local multi-handicapped classroom in high school, which included two days a week at Bittersweet in the horticulture program. His mother was the nurse at Bittersweet, and he adjusted well since he could see his mother daily. His mother reported that Marvin had some natural musical ability and could read simple, single words. Evaluations indicated that Marvin's expressive language was sparse, and his receptive language was a bit more developed. He was hyperactive as a child and was extremely slow motorically when he was admitted. He had extreme lack of initiative. Marvin has a moderate intellectual disability, sensory processing deficits, and an obsessive-compulsive disorder.

Main Problem

Marvin's main problems were his agitation and his self-injurious behaviors of coughing and hard jumping. Marvin jumps very high and brings his knees into his chest. Periods of agitation were generally precipitated by outbursts of temper by other residents. Another problem was compulsive picking which interferes with his ability to develop new skills and participate in activities. Marvin's extreme lack of motivation was a concern.

Unique Approaches and Interventions

In 1999, a psychological report indicated that Marvin continued to exhibit an extreme lack of initiative. He required total supervision to ensure his safety. He needed constant monitoring of important health issues such as proper eating, drinking, and sleeping. Marvin's intake of fluids was critical during hot weather, and he needed prompting for every sip he took. He needed prompting for nearly every activity including going to the bathroom. Interventions at that time were prompts in a variety of modes (verbal, gestural, physical, and pictorial). Due to this problem, Marvin was unable to develop or use skills he may have had in self-care, activities of daily living, and vocational endeavors. In order to decrease Marvin's dependence on verbal prompting and to decrease his self-stimulating and perseverative behaviors, Marvin was scheduled to participate in vigorous activities three times a week, especially hiking and swimming. Physical activities changed with the seasons of the year. Marvin enjoyed the daily hiking and the heavy work of the farm with chopping wood, pushing the wheelbarrow, lifting full buckets of water for the animals, etc. These activities provided Marvin with proprioceptive and vestibular input. They also kept his hands busy so he could not pick. Although one day on a hike he fell behind and was found picking the bark off a tree! A psychological update from 2007 stated that Marvin had an increase in his picking behavior. He picked at his bed until his mattress was torn. When focused on something, he is difficult to redirect. The staff reported that Marvin likes his environment to be perfect. For example, if a door is ajar, he wants to close it or if something is out of place he wants to put it in place. The staff indicated that his obsessive-compulsive behavior had increased, and that there was an increase in wetting his bed. The staff continue to engage Marvin in functional activities, particularly those which promote sensory input.

Marvin's immediate need when he was admitted was communication. He did not initiate speech and, when he was upset, would make a loud throat-clearing noise. Marvin is reminded to look at people before speaking or interacting with them. His vocabulary is enriched throughout the day by the staff using the names of objects and the function and physical attributes of objects. The staff discuss language concepts such as similarities and differences between items. Marvin is encouraged to initiate conversations, and situations are set up to promote conversation. For instance, he is sent on errands to bring things to certain people and then entrusted with a message to return. Marvin worked daily for a period of time with the full-time speech therapist, who in turn, trained the staff on language stimulation.

Based on the program evaluation data, Marvin no longer has problems with aggression and sleep problems. His self-injurious behavior has gone from moderate to mild, as has his anxiety. His limited expressive language was once severe and is now only a moderate problem.

Quality-of-Life Changes

Marvin has made substantial gains in seven of the eight QOL domains. In the domain of self-determination, Marvin has made only mild progress in his ability to be independent. This is due to the fact that Marvin still has challenges in initiative and problem behaviors and needs close supervision. He has endless choices of activities but few personal goals. In the area of personal development, Marvin has made substantial progress in skill development and productivity, but has made only mild gains in personal competence. Marvin demonstrated some natural music ability when he was a child, and at Bittersweet, he participated in the bell choir and had piano and drum lessons taught by the staff. In the domain of physical well-being, Marvin has made substantial gains in self-care skills and hobbies and recreation. Marvin enjoys singing, board games, jigsaw puzzles, crafts, going to church, and looking at magazines. Marvin has made substantial gains in the domains of interpersonal relations and social inclusion. Marvin is quiet and somewhat withdrawn, but now works well with residents and is included in cookouts with the friends with whom he works. Working on art projects and woodworking have given Marvin more opportunities to interact with residents and staff and receive positive responses. Marvin is given many choices and opportunities for meaningful work which could only be provided at a farmstead setting.

Discussion

The partnership aspect of Bittersweet has been critical for Marvin. Partnering with staff in reciprocal activities has helped Marvin become aware of others and to attempt to communicate. He is encouraged to play interactive games such as bingo and puzzles and to read and write with staff. The staff are familiar with Marvin's habits and can protect him from picking up unsafe items and leaving the area without supervision. Marvin may pick up harmful or unsafe items in order to break the object into smaller pieces. Partnership with the staff has also helped Marvin develop positive relationships and friendships which could not occur to this extent in an institution. The active and aerobic focus at Bittersweet encouraged interactive activities with other residents and helped to lessen Marvin's stereotypical autistic behaviors. Marvin enjoys hiking and attending small town fairs. The heavy farm work of pushing, pulling, carrying heavy objects, and mucking the horse stalls has provided Marvin with needed sensory input which helps him calm down The structure of the farmstead allows Marvin to participate in horticulture, wood shop, art studio and groundskeeping. The structure helps motivate Marvin because he is aware of what is expected in each area. All these areas of work provide an enriching environment for Marvin, despite his tendency to withdraw from others. The stimulating, interactive, and active outdoor environment of the farm has allowed Marvin to make significant gains in his quality of life.

Paul

Reason for Admission

Paul has lived at Bittersweet Farms since 2002, although he participated in the day program for several years prior to his residency. His parents were interested in residential placement because Paul's periodic outbursts of anger were becoming more frequent and intense. During one severe episode, Paul, who is 6 feet 7 inches, slapped his mother and squeezed and scratched her hands. Paul was 28 years old at the time of his admission.

Background Information and History

Before moving to Bittersweet Farms, Paul lived with his family and attended special education classes at his public school. In high school, his multi-handicapped classroom was housed at Bittersweet Farms. He has severe autism and a moderate intellectual disability. He has limited communication, self-stimulatory and often ritualistic behavior(s) along with self-injurious episodes. His expressive language is echolalia utterances of two or three words but occasionally occurs in complete sentences. Receptively, he understands the majority of what is said. Paul has sensory processing deficits. Paul was the first transition student at Bittersweet. His school system was not able to manage his aggressive behavior and could not provide adequate educational experiences for him. The school contracted with Bittersweet to have him be part of the day program with a teacher coming out occasionally during the week to monitor his progress. Paul progressed in Bittersweet's classroom setting and was able to enter a special education classroom at his local public high school for the remainder of his education.

Main Problem

Paul had problems with aggression when he came to Bittersweet and would cry for hours at a time. Paul continues to cry, sometimes for extended periods of time, when abrupt and unexplained changes occur in his schedule.

Unique Approaches and Interventions

Exercise and other physical activities have been used to help Paul cope with his sensory processing deficits. Proprioceptive and vestibular deficits were hampering his skill development and were contributing to his agitation. When Paul became a resident, he benefited from the daily hikes and the weekend exercise. Aerobic exercise helps calm Paul down and helps regulate his impulses and behavior. Paul receives sensory input from the heavy work of the farm in lifting, pushing, and pulling activities.

Paul's intervention plan to reduce self-abuse, aggressive behavior, and crying included a number of primary and secondary interventions.

Primary interventions:

1. Provide Paul with a daily schedule and go over it with him in the morning, after lunch, and as he requests throughout the day. If Paul becomes agitated, review his schedule with him.
2. Encourage Paul to verbalize his needs. As tasks are being done, talk to Paul about the task, explaining the steps included to reinforce what he is doing. During breaks, lunch, and other social times, engage in conversation with him, encourage him to answer questions in full sentences and to talk to others. After he has finished a task, go over with him what he accomplished.
3. Provide positive verbal reinforcements frequently, even for small steps of appropriate on-task behavior or other appropriate behaviors.
4. Allow Paul to take short breaks after he has engaged in a task for a sufficient amount of time. If he appears unable to tolerate continuing a task and is getting somewhat agitated, encourage him to complete one more, short step of the task and tell him he can have a break when he is finished.

Secondary interventions:

1. To address crying, have Paul verbalize what's going on with him. At times, he is able to tell you. Go over his schedule with him. If this does not help, it may help to wash his face with cool water, give him a back rub, or take him for a walk. If he does not stop within a few minutes, separate him from the group. Give him ice chips to suck on. Return him to task with positive verbal responses for each small step toward appropriate behavior.

2. To address hitting his face, redirect his hands to his legs or place a pillow between his hands and face. Do not try to physically restrain him, as this agitates him further, and he may view this as a challenge. At times, hitting his face will continue to increase in intensity but remain with him. Either separate him from the group or have the group leave the area. During these periods, it is often helpful to change the staff who are working with Paul.

3. To address aggression toward others, try and react as little as possible, even though at times the kicking or grabbing can be disconcerting. If Paul receives any reaction to his aggressive behavior, he will repeat the same behaviors in order to get the same reaction from that person. If he gets no reaction, he will be much less likely to repeat his aggressive behavior, at least with the same person. Redirect him to another activity without attention to the incident.

A risk assessment rating from 2019 indicated that Paul continues to exhibit some self-injurious behavior on a weekly basis, putting him at risk of medical problems; he has damaged his retinas from slapping himself on the head and face. He may also scratch or gouge his face and neck when extremely agitated. In the past, he would pick his skin in the same spot, often resulting in an open wound. However, this behavior has disappeared. In August 1996, Paul displayed 13 incidents of self-injurious behavior and 7 incidents of grabbing others. Now, he is no longer aggressive. Paul's current goal is to decrease his self-injurious behaviors to an average of five times per month. Paul's problematic behaviors and secondary diagnoses have decreased. His anxiety, depressed mood, and withdrawal once seen by the staff as severe are now viewed as mild. His severe self-injurious behavior is now seen as moderate.

Quality-of-Life Changes

Paul has made substantial gains in five QOL domains. He has made some improvements in all other areas. As a result of the Bittersweet model, Paul has made substantial gains in interpersonal relations and social inclusion. When Paul was an adolescent, his involvement in the community was restricted. His behavior was unpredictable, and he would run and refuse to leave restaurants, stores, etc. His parents were limited to taking him to parks and drive-through restaurants. At times, Paul's parents had to restrain him to control his behavior. Now, Paul participates in small- and large-group activities and attends community activities. Paul now initiates and responds to conversations and can express his needs and interests clearly. He can go shopping and be relaxed and engage in appropriate behaviors. When Paul came to Bittersweet, he could not interact well. Now, he is liked by everyone and has fun with the staff. He loves spelling for people and singing. He has fun repeating commercials, such as: "If it's got to be clean, it's got to be Tide." Paul can repeat the entire Life cereal advertisement with the little boy, Mikey, that ends with "He likes it!! Mikey likes it." The staff love to hear Paul go through this whole routine. In the domain of material well-being, Paul has been given simple but purposeful vocational activities. He seems to be content and to enjoy the activities. In the personal development domain, Paul has made some progress in skill development and personal competence but has substantially improved in his productivity. Paul has only made some improvement in self-care skills and, as a result, has not made substantial improvement in being independent.

Discussion

Paul has significant sensory processing deficits and has benefited from the active and aerobic activities at Bittersweet. He enjoys the hikes, sports, and gross motor activities. Because Paul lives on a farmstead rather than a traditional placement, there are numerous heavy tasks, such as filling large buckets of water and carrying them to the barn to water the animals, cleaning out the horse stalls, and loading the wheelbarrow with wood and pushing it to the wood burning stove in the greenhouse. All these chores provide critical sensory input for Paul, which would not be available in a traditional setting with indoor activities. When he is upset, staff take him for walks or get him involved in an outdoor activity. An outdoor setting has been critical in reducing Paul's aggression and self-injurious behaviors. Paul works best in a consistent and structured environment, and he copes best when he is shown his daily calendar and knows what to expect. The staff show him his calendar multiple times during the day and only show him one month at a time, so he doesn't have to worry about what will be happening in the future.

Working in partnership with the staff has allowed Paul to develop relationships, which give him a sense of community and an awareness of others. In partnership, he has expanded his language skills and can better communicate his needs. Paul is given choices during the day and can explore new vocational interests. Paul has very poor fine motor skills and cannot do tasks that would be available in sheltered workshops or institutions. At Bittersweet, he can do activities outdoors and in the barn. Bittersweet has bird feeders all around the farm, and some are set up so high that Paul, even at 6 feet 7 inches tall, must reach down to get the seed and reach high up to fill the feeders. This helps with flexibility and extending his arms and body. These activities give him confidence and feelings of satisfaction, and lessen his obsessive tendencies. The environment of the farm, with 80 acres and hundreds of different activities available—especially as the seasons change—has helped Paul and other residents to become calm and relaxed. This environment is effective in reducing the stress that tends to trigger aberrant behaviors.

Susan

Reason for Admission

Due to Susan's parents impending divorce in a very stressful family situation and coping with her behavior problems at home, it became necessary to find her a placement. Her mother, along with several other parents and family members led by the founder of Bittersweet Farms, Bettye Ruth Kay, worked very hard for the creation of the facility where young adults (Susan was 23 years at the time) with moderate to severe autism could live in a caring, learning, and safe environment.

Background Information and History

Susan had always lived with her parents and had an early diagnosis of autism and a severe intellectual disability. Susan demonstrated significant behavior problems, including hyperactivity, repetitive and unpredictable screeching, and some hand and body slapping. She would grab at jewelry and people inappropriately and resist following directions. She would be hostile and would bite and scream. She had difficulty with communication, socialization, and pre-academics. Her expressive language was limited, but she knew some sign language, which she did not use. Susan had sensory processing deficits and limited fine motor skills, making it difficult for her to hold silverware or participate in art activities. Susan's strengths were in the self-help area; she could feed and dress herself and disrobe unaided. However, her ability to undress herself became a problem, because she would completely undress and often run around the farm. She would rip up her clothes and, one time, destroyed approximately 100 underpants over the course of a month. Susan was admitted to Bittersweet in 1983 at the age of 22. Evaluations at that time indicated that Susan had a social age of four years.

Main Problem

Susan's aggression was the greatest concern when she arrived at Bittersweet. Her behavior was unpredictable and hostile, and she was

socially inappropriate, often biting and screaming. Agitation would esca-
late into behavioral outbursts which included self-injurious behavior or
aggression.

Unique Approaches and Interventions

Susan responded to the structure the farm provided and the predictable
schedule. Susan did not like to be indoors and engaged in outdoor gross
motor activities which provided sensory input. Initially, a staff member
would accompany her around the farm to see which areas she could participate in. When she was encouraged to participate, she would resist and
throw herself on the floor and have an outburst.

Interventions for reducing Susan's agitation were as follows:

The staff were instructed to provide a full schedule of activities,
including vigorous physical activities, and prepare her for any changes
in routine. When agitation occurred, they would talk to her calmly and
give her the sign to relax. They would then attempt to identify the cause
of her agitation and talk to her about it. Taking her for walks, looking
at picture albums, or letting her take a bath also helped calm her down.

In 1985, two years after Susan's admission to Bittersweet, the staff
viewed her as being able to form attachments, primarily to direct care
staff. Every attempt was made to keep her with consistent staff. Work
assignments were performed with continuous hand-on-hand prompting
because of her extremely short attention span. Her behavior was seen
to have improved dramatically. Her self-injurious behavior was greatly
decreased, destruction of property seldom occurred, and she no long
struck or bit people.

A psychological assessment conducted in 1986 indicated that Susan's
behavior improved after medication helped stabilize her sleep cycles. In
addition, the nurse was able to anticipate pain related to her menstrual
cycles. Her productivity improved and, with close supervision, she could
persist in small uncomplicated tasks, such as shucking corn. The staff
found that Susan performed best with a consistent routine and a stable
environment. The programming was kept routine and the same staff
were assigned to her daily whenever possible.

Quality-of-Life Changes

Despite Susan's significant disabilities, she made substantial gains in all
eight QOL domains. In the domains of interpersonal relations and social
inclusion, the Bittersweet model of partnership helped Susan develop
relationships with a few staff members who were consistently assigned

to her. She was encouraged in her communication skill and began to relate to others. Susan enjoys going swimming and can now go into the community to eat out and shop. In the domain of emotional well-being, Susan expresses a sense of satisfaction and enjoyment in the activities on the farm. Although she does not have many skills, the tasks that the staff find for her are purposeful and provide sensory input. In the domain of rights, Susan is treated with respect and dignity and, as a result, is more comfortable with the staff who partner with her as she works.

Discussion

Susan responds well to the structure, consistency, and flexibility provided at Bittersweet. Allowing Susan to move from one vocational area to another until she finds an area that interests her has been critical.

Farm activities with animals and gross motor tasks allowed her to be productive, where a traditional workshop could not. Susan does not like being inside, and the farm setting allows her to be outdoors and productive. Susan benefits from the aerobic activities that are part of the daily and weekly schedule at Bittersweet. She has severe deficits in fine motor skills and is unable to participate in art projects, but she enjoys walking and hiking. This exercise gives her the sensory input she needs to remain calm. She likes bumpy tractor rides, truck rides, and tearing fabric for weaving. The pulling and resistance in the tearing process activate the receptors in her joints and muscles and provide sensory input. This is a more purposeful activity than tearing her clothes! These activities are not found in traditional residential settings.

The partnership aspect of the Bittersweet model made a great positive impact on Susan. She needed one-on-one supervision when she came to the farm, and all tasks were done in an interactive partnership with the staff. Now, Susan is able to interact with her caretakers and be responsive to other residents. She is now more independent and can move freely around the farm, although she still needs close monitoring. Through partnership, efforts were made to improve her communication, including the use of sign language. The structure of Bittersweet has created a place for Susan to work and interact at her ability level, and experience a much greater quality of life than if she were in a traditional residential placement.

Acknowledgments

I would like to acknowledge the parents on the Board of Bittersweet who desperately wanted this book to be written so that after the original staff retired, the "magic" of the Bittersweet model would not be lost and their children would have continuity in their programming as they aged. I also want to acknowledge Bill Crawford, a Bittersweet parent, who insisted on a Long Range Planning Committee to envision how residents could stay at Bittersweet throughout their lives and what accommodations would make this possible.

Vicki Obee, who was the director of Bittersweet at the start of this project, was critical in getting this project going and added the idea of measuring the Quality of Life impact of the farm on the residents. As Vicki attended meetings around the world, other professionals asked that a research component or program evaluation be included to help make them eligible for government funding.

After Vicki retired, Dustin Watkins became director and continued supporting this project. He supplied the stories and history to help me understand the "magic" I was observing. He provided endless resources and gave me full access to clinical files. Most importantly, he allowed senior staff member, Tammy Chambers, to spend endless time with me. Tammy started to work at Bittersweet in the early 1980s when the residents we studied in the project were admitted as adolescents and young adults. She was instrumental in helping me develop profiles on each of the 20 residents through her stories and understanding of each person's talents and special concerns. Tammy, in her love for the residents, exemplifies what is special about Bittersweet! It is her love, acceptance, and relationship with each resident that demonstrates the family-like feeling the residents experience with Tammy and each staff member.

Carol Quick started this project and used her fabulous writing skills and creativity to develop a framework that used examples and stories which allows the book to be read by a wide audience of parents, staff, and academics. Ruth Wilson, PhD, writer, editor, and book developer, brought the book to completion and added the critical research on the impact of environment on people with autism which is central to understanding the farmstead model and the appropriateness of this treatment program.

Nancy Buderer, biostatistician, research consultant, and program evaluator, developed a Quality of Life scale to measure the difference in quality of life indices of residents when they came to Bittersweet until the present time. This allowed us to measure the impact of the Bittersweet model and conclude, as the parents thought, that it really was "magical" and greatly benefited the residents. Thank you, Nancy, for helping us enrich our study by adding this dimension to our analysis.

I want to thank Kathryn Dennler, PhD, scholar and researcher, who gave me invaluable help in analyzing data and formulating conclusions.

Kim Manrigue, art therapist, contributed many graphic designs for the book as well as providing art therapy and design consultation. Thank you, Kim!

Sarah Kieswetter Boerst, a former Bittersweet employee and occupational therapist, spent hours and even a weekend in northern Michigan to help me further understand the components of the model and the complexities of the individual residents. I learned how the farmstead setting and the various activities helped calm the residents and reduce their sensory problems which were so intense in other settings. Addressing the sensory needs of each individual is key to improving their adjustment and allowing them to be productive and interactive, thus increasing their quality of life.

I want to acknowledge Temple Grandin, author, for calling me back and taking interest in Bittersweet Farms, which she had visited many years before. She asked to read sections of the book and gave excellent feedback and direction. It was my great pleasure to work with her and receive her support and guidance!

While writing this book and collecting data for the program evaluation, I spent hours on the farm interviewing staff and residents and watching them all, in partnership, do the work on the farm. There were moments I will never forget seeing the kindness, patience, and respectful way the staff interacted with the residents. One parent I interviewed pondered how Bittersweet could attract such wonderful staff who treated her daughter as family, often including her in their family's parties and special occasions. I think that must just be the essence of Bittersweet which you can feel when you drive in and get out of your car to have a resident welcome you and offer you a tour. There is just something about being at the farmstead which operates at a slow but steady pace on 80 acres of beautiful farmland and woods. I want to thank all the staff who have ever worked at the farm and those to come for caring for the residents and improving their quality of life.

Jeanne Dennler, PhD

Index

For Product Safety Concerns and Information please contact our EU
representative GPSR@taylorandfrancis.com
Taylor & Francis Verlag GmbH, Kaufingerstraße 24, 80331 München, Germany

www.ingramcontent.com/pod-product-compliance
Ingram Content Group UK Ltd.
Pitfield, Milton Keynes, MK11 3LW, UK
UKHW021425080625
459435UK00011B/167